100 Weight Loss Tips & Stop Dieting

100 Weight Loss Tips & How to Stop Dieting and Eat Normally

By Nicholas Bjorn

Nicholas Bjorn

Weight Loss

100 Weight Loss Tips
Lose Weight and Maintain Healthy Weight Loss through Diet, Exercise and Lifestyle

3rd Edition

By Nicholas Bjorn

Nicholas Bjorn

© Copyright 2015 – 2019 by Nicholas Bjorn – All rights reserved.

The contents of this book may not be reproduced, duplicated, or transmitted without direct written permission from the author.

Under no circumstances will any legal responsibility or blame be held against the publisher for any reparation, damages, or monetary loss due to the information herein, either directly or indirectly.

Legal Notice:

This book is copyright protected. This is only for personal use. You cannot amend, distribute, sell, use, quote, or paraphrase any part of the content within this book without the consent of the author.

Disclaimer Notice:

Please note the information contained within this document is for educational and entertainment purposes only. Every attempt has been made to provide accurate, up-to-date, complete, and reliable information. No warranties of any kind are expressed or implied. Readers acknowledge that the author is not engaging in the rendering of legal, financial, medical, or professional advice. The content of this book has been derived from various sources. Please consult a licensed professional before attempting any techniques outlined in this book.

By reading this document, the reader agrees that under no circumstances is the author responsible for any losses, direct or indirect, which are incurred as a result of the use of information contained within this document, including, but not limited to, errors, omissions, or inaccuracies.

Nicholas Bjorn

Table of Contents

Introduction 15

Chapter 1 – Benefits of Losing Weight 17

    1. Diabetes and Prediabetes Prevention 17

    2. Makes You Heart Healthy 18

    3. Improved Sleep by Reducing Snoring 18

    4. Pain-free Joints 18

    5. Improved Energy 19

    6. You Feel Better 19

Chapter 2 – 40 Diet Tips to Lose Weight 21

    1. Create a Grocery List 21

    2. Shop the Perimeter of the Grocery Store 24

    3. Include Whole Foods, and Cut Down on Processed Foods 25

    4. Curb Your Sweet Tooth Naturally 27

    5. Slow Down and Hara Hachi Bu Rule 28

    6. Do Not Completely Eliminate Carbohydrates 28

    7. Increase Consumption of Fruits and Vegetables 29

    8. Choose Grilled Food over Fried 29

    9. Increase Fiber Intake 31

10.	Be Conscious of Your Calorie Intake	31
11.	Increase Water Intake	32
12.	Use Your Utensils Carefully	32
13.	Have Occasional Treats	32
14.	Learn to Cook Delicious Food and Invest in Equipment 33	
15.	Plan Out and Shop for Snacks	34
16.	Healthy Recipes	34
17.	Distinct Journals	35
18.	Jot it Down	35
19.	Curb Those Cravings	36
20.	Be Prepared, Be Ready	37
21.	Throw Away the Junk	37
22.	Low-calorie Meals and Tasty Smoothies	38
23.	Never Skip Breakfast	38
24.	Eat This, Not That	39
25.	Measure Up!	40
26.	Breakfast Made Healthy	40
27.	Healthy Soup and Preparation of the Day	41
28.	Cut the Calories	42
29.	Swap It!	44

30. Desserts and How to Make Them Healthy 45

31. Snacks and How to make them Healthy 46

32. Reduce the Size of Your Plate 47

33. Chewing Gum All the Time 47

34. Low Salt, Less Butter 48

35. Go Meatless Once a Week 48

36. Cut It Out 48

37. Think and Eat 49

38. Drink Your Coffee Black 49

39. Eat Your Dinner Early 50

40. Be Patient 52

Chapter 3 – 20 Exercise Tips to Lose Weight 55

1. Commit to a Set Amount of Time 55

2. Build a Workout Routine 56

3. Set a Schedule for Your Workouts 61

4. Try High-intensity Interval Workouts 62

5. Power Up Your Run 63

6. Switch It Up 63

7. Use High-quality Clothes While Working Out 64

8. Find a Workout Partner 64

9. Choose Your Tunes 65

10.	Pay Attention to Your Form	65
11.	Do Compound Exercises	66
12.	Use the Body that You Have	66
13.	Accept Discomfort	67
14.	Try Something New	68
15.	Don't Forget to Rest	70
16.	Realize that You Can't Do it Alone	70
17.	New Rewards	71
18.	Track Your Body	72
19.	Watch Your Clothes	73
20.	Patience	74

Chapter 4 – 20 Lifestyle Tips for Weight Loss............77

1.	Change Your Mindset	77
2.	Make It a Commitment, and Write It Down	78
3.	Document Your Weight Loss	78
4.	Morning Routine	79
5.	Predefined Hours	82
6.	Find Your Motivation	83
7.	Plan a SMART Goal	84
8.	Sharing is Caring	85
9.	Get a Sipper	85

10.	Change Your Eating Habits	85
11.	Don't Follow Crazy Diets	86
12.	Walk and Talk	89
13.	Do Not Focus Too Much on the Scale	89
14.	Make It Fun	90
15.	Use Tools and Gadgets to Help You	91
16.	Learn to Celebrate Each Accomplishment	91
17.	Put Your Excuses Away	92
18.	Tackling Necessary Restaurant Visits	92
19.	Patience Matters	95
20.	Understand the Reason	96

Chapter 5 – 20 Tips to Maintain Weight Loss 97

1.	Write Down Why Your Goals Matter	97
2.	Create Goals for the Week	98
3.	Chain Your Events and Goals	99
4.	Follow a Consistent Routine	100
5.	Use a Plan that Works for You	101
6.	Follow Your Plan	101
7.	Stay Active	102
8.	Don't Skip Days	103
9.	Keep Stress at Bay	104

10.	Sleep Well	105
11.	Avoid Unplanned Eating and Drinking	105
12.	Plan and Set Reminders	105
13.	Make Sure You Have a Healthy Perspective on Food	106
14.	Maintain a Positive Mindset	106
15.	Fuel Your Body Before and After Workouts	107
16.	Be Inspired; Don't Compare	107
17.	Words Can Be Inspiring	109
18.	Imagine Your Success	110
19.	Compete with the Past You	111
20.	Be Patient	113

Chapter 6 – 12 Bonus Recipes to Get on with Your Diet 115

Pizza Crust Made of Quinoa 115

Creamy Thai Soup 117

Green Pea and Parsley Soup 118

Stuffed Sweet Potatoes 119

Baked Paleo Chicken 121

Brunch Banana Pancakes 123

Hawaiian Chicken Salad 124

Vegan Risotto 126

Moo Shu Beef 128

Amaranth salad 130

Risotto Soup 132

Tuna Salad 133

Conclusion 135

Nicholas Bjorn

Introduction

Thank you for choosing my latest book, *"Weight Loss: 100 Weight Loss Tips: Lose Weight and Maintain Healthy Weight Loss through Diet, Exercise and Lifestyle."* With this book, you will learn exactly what you need to start doing today to lose weight and what it takes to reach your weight loss goals.

This book contains proven steps and strategies on how to successfully lose weight. There are a lot of good reasons to lose excess weight. Over the past few years, obesity has become known as the main risk factor for diseases like diabetes and heart ailments. It can also affect your quality of life and prevent you from doing some of the activities that you used to enjoy.

Weight loss can be achieved by changing some aspects of your lifestyle, especially your diet and level of physical activity. This book contains diet, exercise, and lifestyle tips that can motivate you to lose weight. However, you shouldn't stop once you achieve your ideal weight. Maintaining your weight loss also has its own challenges. The last chapter of this book provides some tips on how you can maintain your weight and lose some more.

Thanks again for choosing this book, and I hope you enjoy it!

Nicholas Bjorn

FREE E-BOOKS SENT WEEKLY

Join North Star Readers Book Club
And Get Exclusive Access To The Latest Kindle Books in Health, Fitness, Weight Loss and Much More…

TO GET YOU STARTED HERE IS YOUR FREE E-BOOK:

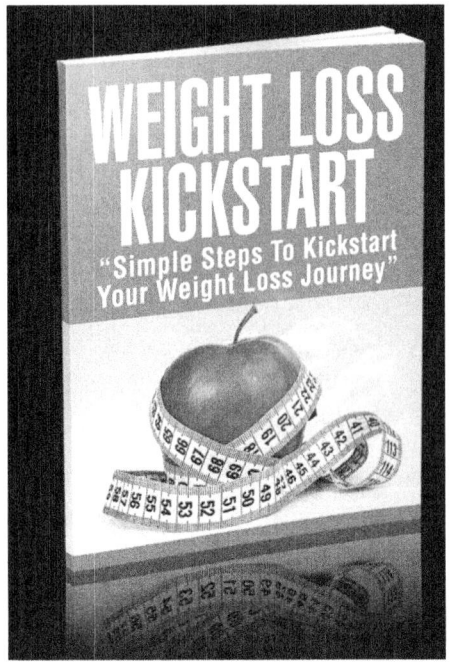

Visit to Sign Up Today!
www.northstarreaders.com/weight-loss-kick-start

Chapter 1 – Benefits of Losing Weight

Weight loss is one of the most popular topics in magazines, lifestyle talk shows, and even normal conversation. There are a lot of people who dedicate their lives to helping people achieve their weight goals. Oftentimes, weight loss is considered as the effect of pop culture and social media, which cultivate images of the "perfect" body. However, losing weight has a lot of short-term and long-term benefits. These benefits are definitely worth the patience and hard work necessary to lose weight.

1. Diabetes and Prediabetes Prevention

Prediabetes occurs when the body has blood glucose that is higher than normal but not high enough to be diagnosed as diabetes. Type 2 diabetes occurs when the body doesn't produce enough insulin to function properly. Having prediabetes can place a person at a higher risk of developing diabetes in the future.

Obesity is one of the major risk factors of type 2 diabetes. It can be difficult for the body's cells to respond to insulin if it carries excess weight. Fat cells act like a wall that prevents sugar from entering the cells, thus resulting in a higher blood sugar level. Studies show that even just a weight loss of 7% through a combination of diet and exercise can prevent prediabetes by 60%.

2. Makes You Heart Healthy

The major risk factors of heart disease are high cholesterol and high blood pressure. Accumulation of excess body fat can cause blood pressure to increase and can trigger the liver to produce high amounts of cholesterol. Losing weight will reduce your blood pressure, along with reducing the amount of cholesterol in your body.

3. Improved Sleep by Reducing Snoring

Snoring happens when the airways are constricted, consequently producing the basic characteristics of a "snore." People who carry excess weight tend to have excess tissue in their neck. This excess tissue increases the chances of snoring and can also lead to a serious and life-threatening condition known as sleep apnea. This condition occurs when the airway is obstructed and the person has to wake up to breathe again. Losing weight reduces the total amount of fat in the body, including that in the neck. Maintaining a healthy weight also improves sleep quality. People who are fit and slim sleep well and have deeper sleep and a wonderful sleep cycle. Such people also have less nightmares, and they wake up feeling refreshed.

4. Pain-free Joints

Excess weight can place strain on your joints, which consequently become swollen and tender. Movement can be very difficult if you have a joint disorder. Even a weight loss of 5% of your total body weight can significantly reduce the amount of stress on your hips, knees, and back. Weight loss can also increase your standing time, as you can stand for longer times if you lose weight. This is great for teachers and professors who are supposed to stand up a lot. It won't have much of a negative effect.

5. Improved Energy

Losing weight through regular exercise can enhance your strength and vitality. Moderate workouts in the morning can help keep you energized throughout the day. This is a great benefit for people who often find themselves sleepy after lunch. Weight loss makes you highly active as well. You feel fresh, active, and peppy throughout the day. You can finish heavy tasks in less time without feeling tired. A sort of different aura will surround you, which will also make you appear more positive and radiant because of weight loss.

6. You Feel Better

Losing weight can naturally make you feel better. The extra weight that you carry in your stomach can squeeze the kidney and prevent it from processing toxins, which can make you feel sluggish. You will also feel lighter and more confident. Exercise releases hormones that are responsible for making you feel good. Losing weight and achieving a healthy body can also boost your self-confidence. You will start to realize that you are capable of accomplishing your goals, which will make you feel more confident about your skills. All of this happens because subconsciously people develop a negative image of themselves when they are overweight. Partly, society is to blame for this. However, when you lose weight, you definitely start feeling more confident and attractive. Use this new power to keep yourself well maintained and to prevent the weight and fats from coming back.

Chapter 2 – 40 Diet Tips to Lose Weight

Watching what you eat is one of the best ways to successfully lose weight. Dieting has become very popular recently and still is gaining a lot of popularity. However, not all diets are healthy; some of them are actually fad diets that may help you lose weight in less time, but these diets will actually cause more problems than benefits. These diets are famous for quick weight loss, so people tend to ignore their side effects. Unfortunately, some of the side effects of such diets can actually prove to be fatal. Weight loss is important but not more important than your life; do not forget that.

However, the above statement does not mean that you cannot use dieting to lose weight–you surely can–but instead of relying on fad diets or crash diets, you should ideally consult you GP or a good dietician who can help you to formulate a good diet plan according to your body and health. If you do not want to go to a doctor or a dietician, you can always find some really great diet options online, but remember not to look for fad or crash diets. Weight loss is supposed to be a long process because sudden weight loss may actually cause many problems.

Here are some foods and diet tips that can help you lose weight.

1. Create a Grocery List

Eating healthy is a very crucial part of the weight loss process. You have to keep this in mind and stock up on healthy food accordingly. You cannot pick up random foods from the grocery aisles anymore. Make a grocery list before you visit the store. This will allow you to stay on track and help you avoid any unhealthy purchases. You have to make conscious choices about what you eat if you want to lose weight.

A grocery list will help you with this. We all tend to prepare our meals with whatever is at hand at home. This means that you will be preparing healthy meals if you stock up on healthy ingredients. However, if you buy bags of chips and cookies, you will most likely be reaching for them at some point in the day.

Instead, you can create a grocery list that includes nutrient-rich food that will benefit your body, and only buy these on your next grocery store run. Instead of sugar-laden cookies, add some whole grain crackers to your list. These kinds of switches in your grocery list will make a lot of difference in what you consume in the long run. Buy nutritious foods that will fit into your weight loss plan.

The following are some of the foods you should include in your healthy grocery list:

- Whole grains like brown rice, buckwheat groats, whole-wheat pasta or tortillas, and whole grain bread.

- Fruits like papaya, kiwi, cantaloupe, strawberries, blueberries, avocado, oranges, apples, bananas, honeydew melon, and grapes.

- Vegetables like acorn squash, spinach, Swiss chard, red peppers, red lettuce, tomatoes, onions, broccoli, garlic, ginger, lemons, cilantro, and carrots.

- Beans and legumes like pinto beans, white beans, green beans, and garbanzo beans.

- Fish like salmon, king mackerel, trout, and Bluefin tuna.

- Dairy and soy foods like nonfat milk, soy yogurt, reduced-fat cheddar cheese, soy turkey, soy cheese, soybeans, and eggs.

- Nuts, seeds, and foods like olive oil, almonds, tahini, and walnuts.

- Condiments like salt, pepper, ground cumin, Italian dressing, maple syrup, vegetable broth, chicken broth, balsamic vinegar, red wine vinegar, cinnamon, honey mustard, salsa, and cornstarch.

All of the above are foods that usually fit into any healthy diet. So, the next time you grab a cart at the grocery store, stick to foods that are only included in your list. Avoid loading up on anything that you will feel guilty about eating later.

Meal planning is a great idea when you want to have greater control over your diet. It involves planning out all your meals for a week or more. Then, you can prepare most of the ingredients and even prepare the food and keep it ready for consumption. The dishes will be portioned out so that you have food ready for all your meals. Some of the dishes can be half-cooked, or you can just keep the ingredients ready for you to cook when you actually want to eat. The point is that you can start meal prepping to help you with weight loss. While you decide on the dishes you want for the week, check out the recipes that are given later in the book. It will give you an idea about the kind of food you can eat while trying to lose weight.

Recipes will have ingredient lists, and these can be of great help. Note down all the ingredients you will require to prepare all the food. This will be your weekly grocery list. You can mindfully buy things that you will be using during the week while staying away from other potentially fattening food. This will save you a lot of time and serve as another great way to do better on your weight loss plan.

You can keep trying new dishes that are suitable for your goals while enjoying your food without worrying about gaining weight. A thorough grocery list before you go shopping will save you a lot of stress and time for the next week or so. Everything you need and should be eating will be stocked up in the house. Remember to get rid of the unhealthy food in your pantry that might set you adrift from your goals.

2. Shop the Perimeter of the Grocery Store

Even when you go to the grocery store, there is a right way and a wrong way to be shopping. Most of us mindlessly wander around the grocery store and pick up whatever we want. It has also been noticed that people have a tendency to shop more from the aisles in the center. If you think about it, you will usually walk straight into the center when you enter a store. However, if you want to eat healthier, you should be shopping at the perimeters of your local grocery store. Typically, the healthiest foods are at the back or the outer sides of the grocery store.

Most of the fresh food will be stocked in this area. Fresh foods like produce, dairy, or meat are generally kept in the perimeter region of most grocery stores and should be what you buy more of. These foods are much healthier than the processed foods that you generally buy from the center aisles. The center aisles are stocked to the brim with tons of options, but all of this is processed and unhealthy food. You don't need to buy varieties of cookies and chips just because they taste good and there are always new flavors to try.

The modern diet is filled with this kind of junk food, and this is why most of us suffer from weight issues. The availability of these processed foods has made things a lot more convenient, but this comes at the cost of our health. Buying fresh produce is always the better choice, even if it takes up time to cook your own meals. It allows you to have a lot more control over how much fat and sodium you consume in your diet. It is important for you to take notice of what is added to your food if you want to maintain a healthy diet.

Processed foods usually have a lot of preservatives that do more harm and good in the long run. Such ingredients allow manufacturers to increase the shelf life of their food products. However, there are chemicals and hidden additives that have a negative effect on your body. A packet of chips can lie on the shelf for months together, while fruits and vegetables have to be switched out every few days.

In their natural state and without preservatives, food tends to spoil quite easily. However, these wholesome fresh foods are what your body needs. You need to fill your kitchen with baskets of fresh fruits, and the fridge should only have vegetables and fresh meat. The processed meals and condiments have minimal nutrition and a ton of calories to add to your weight. So, opt for as much of the fresh foods from the perimeters as possible, and avoid the central aisles when you go grocery shopping again. The added benefit is that you will also be saving a lot of money while you do this.

3. Include Whole Foods, and Cut Down on Processed Foods

Like we mentioned above, it is important to eat more whole foods and less processed foods. A diet that is rich in whole foods is more likely to help you lose weight over time. This is because whole foods are usually much closer to their natural state than any processed food.

Processed foods will have a lot of additives, such as sugar, salt, starch, flavorings, and other things that will actually cause an increase in weight and even harm your health. They have certain substances that allow manufacturers to keep them on the shelves longer, but these substances are harmful to the human body. Whole foods are more nutritious and allow you to eat clean. They won't have hidden ingredients that you have to worry about. Eating whole foods gives you more control over what you put in your body.

For instance, opt for potatoes from the produce section, and avoid buying potato chips from processed foods. Buy a whole chicken, and grill it for lunch instead of eating chicken nuggets. Check the labels of the foods you purchase, and avoid foods that are overly processed. They will be filled with preservatives and artificial ingredients while barely providing any nutrition. You might be a little unsure about what is processed and what is considered a whole food, so the following should help you out:

- Whole foods include fresh fruits, vegetables, milk, nuts, seeds, meat, poultry, beans, and seafood.
- Processed foods include ready-to-eat meals, refined carbohydrates, foods that have added sugars, junk food, and anything that is highly processed.

When you are buying fruits and vegetables, try to get the freshest variety. Canned or frozen foods should be consumed only if there are minimal additives added. Packaged fruit juices are processed and usually filled with sugars, but making juice from the real fruit will be a wholesome option. It would also be a better option to soak beans at home before preparing them instead of buying canned beans.

Milk itself is a whole food, but dairy products are processed to a certain level. Buy minimally processed cheese and yogurt. Be careful about the meat or poultry you buy as well because some varieties contain a lot of hormones and antibiotics that you should preferably avoid. Ready-to-eat foods may save you time, but they are not healthy and cause weight gain. Prepare meals from scratch for better nutrition and taste. Foods with refined carbohydrates are processed and should be avoided. This includes puffed rice and anything that is made from white flour. When grains are ground into flour, they become more glycemic. Opt for barley, quinoa, or brown rice.

4. Curb Your Sweet Tooth Naturally

Sweet treats like candies, cakes, and cookies are very delicious and appetizing, but they are loaded with artificial ingredients that do not provide much benefit for the body. Additionally, these sugary foods can have negative effects on the body. These treats have high calories and thus make it easier for you to gain weight. They can also trigger blood sugar fluctuations that can cause mood swings.

However, it is also unrealistic and unreasonable to remove all sweet foods from your diet completely. Fruits are called "nature's candy" because of their natural sweetness. Unlike candies, fruits contain fiber, vitamins, and minerals that can provide many benefits for the body. Keep a stash of fruit in your kitchen so that you won't be tempted to overindulge in processed sweets when you have a craving.

5. Slow Down and Hara Hachi Bu Rule

It takes about 20 minutes for the body to realize that you are already full. Eating mindlessly can make you eat more calories than you need. Take time to enjoy your meals. It is better if you eat on a table instead of in front of the television because watching can distract you from enjoying your meal. Take your time, and eat slowly. A study at the University of Rhode Island showed that a person can lose about 2 pounds a month if they eat slowly because they become more aware of what they are consuming.

You should also avoid eating too much food until you are stuffed full. Overeating can make it uncomfortable for you to move or even breathe afterwards. There is a practice in Japan known as "hara hachi bu" where you should eat only until you feel that you are 80% full. Do undertake this practice, and avoid eating until you get full. According some Indian traditions, you should divide your stomach into three parts. So, fill half of your stomach with food, a quarter with water, and a quarter with air.

6. Do Not Completely Eliminate Carbohydrates

Carbohydrates have been labeled as one of the causes of weight gain. However, the real reason behind its bad reputation is that most of the carbohydrates that people consume are highly processed. If a standard diet of eating processed carbs and one that is low in carbohydrates are compared, it looks like the latter wins in terms of being the best way to lose weight. However, the results are different if the low-carbohydrate diet is compared with a good carb diet that is low in processed foods and sugars.

Before 1991, Japanese people made carbohydrates part of their regular meals. They often eat rice and sweet potatoes, but they are considered one of the healthiest people in the world. Obesity is uncommon in Japan, unlike the case in other countries. The body needs adequate carbohydrates to function well. Completely removing carbohydrates from your diet can affect the hormones responsible for fat loss and consequently make it harder for you to lose weight. As a general rule, eat more carbohydrates on days in which you expect to be more physically active.

7. Increase Consumption of Fruits and Vegetables

People who eat more fruits and vegetables are healthier and slimmer than those who constantly eat processed foods. Fruits and vegetables are rich in nutrients that can give you energy. Moreover, these foods are free from sugars and artificial ingredients, which can be toxic to the body. Aim to eat different colored vegetables and fruits. Fortunately, fruits and vegetables are delicious and versatile, so you can add them to your dishes easily.

8. Choose Grilled Food over Fried

The way you cook your food will have a big impact on the quality of your diet and its effect on your weight loss plan. It is a healthier option to grill food than fry them. Frying involves a lot of oil or fat, and this can cause weight gain. It may be tempting to eat such fried foods because they taste and smell good, but they are not going to help you lose weight. Instead, you can switch over to grilling most of the foods that you usually fry. They will taste good, and you will also have the satisfaction of knowing that you are eating healthy.

Nicholas Bjorn

Fried foods cause high calorie intake, and it results in unwanted weight gain. If you opt to cook most of your food by frying, it will be more difficult to manage your weight. In fact, a lot of nutrition is lost from certain foods when they are fried. The high temperature of the fat or oil that you fry the food with will result in moisture loss and will cause vitamins to be eliminated. Fried foods are also much harder to digest than grilled foods. You need to eat food that can be digested well and not stored as fat.

Any food that has a very high fat content will exert too much pressure on your digestive system and can cause health issues. Grilling is a healthier cooking method with many benefits. When you grill meat, it will have reduced fat when you eat it. This is because a lot of fat will melt off the meat while grilling. It will allow you to consume a diet that is much lower in fat content. The calorie content of grilled food is also lower than that of fried food. Your calorie consumption will be much more controlled, and this will promote better weight management.

Eating more grilled food will also help you achieve lower levels of bad cholesterol in your body. Fried food increases bad cholesterol and affects cardiovascular health. Changing your method of cooking will reduce your risk of developing conditions like type 2 diabetes, stroke, high blood pressure, etc. Grilling will ensure that your food is much more nutritious, thus improving your overall health while helping you lose excess weight. It will prevent moisture loss from your food and also retain the vitamins you need.

Many people don't know that grilling food allows vegetables to retain more vitamins and minerals than frying does. Grilling is especially better for vegetables that already have low water content because it allows them to retain moisture. Another advantage is that the vegetables that are usually chosen for grilling are fresh and in season. This is a better alternative to canned veggies and will aid in your weight loss plan.

When you grill a slab of meat over a fire, it will preserve more of its thiamine and riboflavin. These have their own health benefits and play a vital role in the diet. Once you master the process of grilling your food, you will always opt for it over frying. Given that grilled food retains more moisture, you will also be less inclined to add any fattening condiments like butter to your food. This means that your meals will have fewer calories. Opt for lean meats to grill because they will give you more protein and less fat. No matter what you cook, grilling is the way to do it. Healthy cooking will contribute to better weight management.

9. Increase Fiber Intake

Increasing your fiber intake can encourage weight loss by making you feel full even if you consume fewer calories. Eating fiber-rich foods like whole grains, whole produce, and beans can also reduce your cravings, making you less likely to binge on unhealthy foods later in the day.

10. Be Conscious of Your Calorie Intake

Consuming fewer calories than what you burn is the most straightforward way to lose weight. Your ideal calorie intake depends on your current weight, height, and level of physical activity. There are calorie calculators online that automatically calculate these numbers. You can easily reduce your calorie intake by consuming less processed food and focusing on nourishing your body with whole food. However, you should also refrain from eating very few calories because this can be detrimental to your health. As you lose weight, you should adjust your calorie budget accordingly because you will need fewer calories as your body becomes lighter.

11. Increase Water Intake

Drinking water has numerous benefits, including detoxification and suppressing your appetite. There are times when you confuse thirst for hunger. Drinking water can help you reduce your food intake and make you feel fuller. It also reduces water retention in the body, which can help you lose a lot of water weight. Water should be your choice of beverage rather than high-calorie sodas and juices.

12. Use Your Utensils Carefully

You can eat less by using different utensils and plates when eating. By simply using a smaller plate, you can trick your brain into thinking that you are consuming more food. This rule also applies to drinks. Tall and lean drinking glasses are better than short and wide ones. Some people also opt to use chopsticks instead of a spoon and fork to help them eat more slowly.

13. Have Occasional Treats

Having the perfect diet that eliminates all kinds of unhealthy food is unrealistic. Aiming for perfection can be counterproductive because it can make you feel deprived and depressed. It is okay to indulge in your favorite treats every once in a while. A few scoops of ice cream and one slice of cake will not hurt your diet. However, be careful not to make these occasional treats a regular indulgence. Aim to have treats comprise 10% to 15% of your total diet. This way, you will not feel deprived.

14. Learn to Cook Delicious Food and Invest in Equipment

Relying on restaurant food can be detrimental to your health and budget. Invest in a good cookbook, and start cooking on your own. Learning how to cook can be fun and exciting. You will also feel a sense of accomplishment after preparing dishes that you and your family can enjoy. Cooking your own food can enable you to control your ingredients and serving sizes.

You should also invest in kitchen equipment to make cooking easier. If you often lack time to cook at home, you can purchase a slow cooker so that you can simply prepare the ingredients ahead of time and come home to a warm cooked meal in the evening. A slow cooker is also very versatile and economical because it consumes less electricity than an oven.

A food processor and blender are also great tools to use. You can make fruit shakes and green smoothies using a blender. Such shakes and smoothies are great alternatives to whole vegetables and fruits. Finally, store your leftovers in the freezer after cooking a large batch of food. Freezing the food can maintain freshness and preserve nutrients. You can also buy a large bulk of fresh vegetables and fruits that are on sale and then freeze them to prolong their shelf life.

15. Plan Out and Shop for Snacks

A properly devised and developed exercise and diet routine is extremely essential for anyone who wants to lose weight. Without a proper plan, your hard work may not benefit you at all. Everyone loves snacks, and people who love food are generally reluctant about dropping their favorite snacks. Unfortunately, most of these generally loved snacks are fatty and unhealthy. However, you do not need to drop your snacks altogether; you just need to reduce your intake of these snacks. It is also advisable to plan out your snacks once a week. This preplanning is always helpful and will prevent binge eating or unhealthy eating.

16. Healthy Recipes

Generally, everyone loves food but more often than not, all of us love foods that are considered to be fatty and very unhealthy. Instead of eating these fatty and unhealthy foods, you should opt for healthy and nutritious foods. It is a very popular myth that healthy and nutritious food does not taste good. This is a lie. Nutritious and healthy food can be very tasty if you follow good and well-tested recipes. You can find such recipes online. These recipes will make you fall in love with healthy food. You can also buy recipe books that are specially made for people who want to lose weight. These recipes are well researched so they will not have any side effects.

If you have some health problems, you should ideally consult with your dietician or doctor first about recipes. Your dietician can prescribe and suggest the best recipes for you.

17. Distinct Journals

In the next few chapters, you will find that I have mentioned a lot about keeping journals. Keeping at least two journals concerning your diet is highly necessary. The personal journal will be explained in the next chapters, but here, we will talk about the public journal. Keeping a public journal that you can share with the public or friends is a very good way to keep yourself motivated. As the public will check your progress every day, you will feel a sense of responsibility, as well as a challenge to do well. This responsibility and challenge will lead you to results faster.

You can keep a public journal in many ways, of which two are extremely common and easy to do. You can send an e-copy of your journal every night to your friends through email. Another option is posting your progress in online forums for weight loss. These two options will help you a lot. You should always keep one thing in mind though; you should always fill in correct details and information in your journal, as wrong information can ruin your diet plan. Remember, honesty is the best policy for losing weight.

18. Jot it Down

Keep a big white board or chalkboard in your kitchen, and jot down your total diet plan on this board. Jotting down your diet plan and keeping it in focus all the time will keep you motivated and accountable. This constant reminder will keep you active and peppy. You should also jot down your weekly meal plan on the board so that you can follow the plan thoroughly. By making a weekly plan, you can keep a track of your daily calories and nutrients easily.

Another benefit of keeping a white board or chalkboard is that you can write beautiful inspirational and motivational quotes on it. Although motivational quotes have faced a lot of ridicule in recent times, this does not mean they are useless. You can feel the change if you keep yourself motivated. Remember, losing weight is not just about physical strength; it is also about mental strength and mind power. If you keep yourself motivated, the journey of weight loss will not be hard at all.

19. Curb Those Cravings

One of the biggest if not **the** biggest enemy of your weight loss journey is craving. Human beings are heavy gluttons—we love food. It's not a hyperbole if someone says that we live to eat not eat to live. Unfortunately, diet is all about controlling your intake of calories, which means controlling your intake of food as well. However, as human beings, we cannot control ourselves when we are on restrictions to eat food.

Curbing the cravings is not much of an issue if you are full all the time. This can be achieved by eating foods that are rich in fiber and are filling. Another major problem with cravings is that sometimes you get cravings even when you are full. You need to understand that these cravings are not actually cravings but just boredom or emotional pain. People eat food when they feel sad, frustrated, angry, or even when they are bored. To overcome these cravings, you should try doing things that will kill your boredom or will help you to overcome your pain, sadness, depression, tension, anger, etc. These activities may include chatting with a close friend, going out for a walk, taking a bath, sleeping, reading your favorite book, etc. Doing yoga and some breathing exercises are also good options.

20. Be Prepared, Be Ready

Hunger can strike anytime, anywhere. It is highly necessary to address your cravings effectively. You should not eat high fatty foods etc to curb your cravings. You should ideally keep cut fruits and veggies in your refrigerator for emergency cravings. Cut-up fruits and veggies are not only effective in curbing the cravings, but you can also arrange a quick snack or cook a small but healthy meal instantly with these sliced and diced veggies and fruits.

21. Throw Away the Junk

It has already been established that human beings love food, especially junk food. Keeping junk food in the house, especially in places that can be reached easily, is a massive problem. You keep on going back to your junk food because human beings simply cannot control their desires for too long if their prey sits smugly in front of them. We succumb to such desires, which are quite natural, but this should be avoided at all costs.

To overcome this problem, it is advisable to throw out all the junk food from your house. Now, this is quite easy if you are a bachelor or spinster, but it might become a nuisance for people who have roommates or live with their family, partner, spouse, etc. For such people, the only option is to make the others understand that snacking can be a very big hindrance to your diet and exercise regime, and so to help you, they should keep off the snacks for a bit. If this does not work (and there are a lot of chances of this happening), you can try asking them to buy small amounts of snacks at a time, which can be eaten in one go or, at most, two go's. This will definitely help you avoid snacks.

37

22. Low-calorie Meals and Tasty Smoothies

This tip might be very hard to follow as people love to eat, as already established in this book a few times. Reducing your meal to such a simple affair of 300 to 400 calories is a hard thing to do, especially if you are accustomed to heavy meals and unhealthy foods. You will probably feel irritated, frustrated, and sometimes downright angry if you simply try to shift to a diet with meals consisting of just 300 to 400 calories. You can obviously tolerate this kind of diet and prevent these sorts of side effects if you plan your diet properly. Instead of eating 40 calories of ice cream or something of that sort, you should concentrate hard on including foodstuffs that are low on calories but still highly fulfilling. These things will help you feel satiated quite easily and quickly without consuming a lot of calories. Moreover, these calories are not the so-called empty calories.

There are certain options that are supposed to be really fulfilling as well. These options include healthy and tasty smoothies. You can make tasty smoothies and add healthy ingredients, such as avocados, greens, berries, etc. These things will revamp your smoothies and will make them even more healthy and delicious.

Remember, 300 to 400 calories do not have to be a bad thing if you manage your diet well. You will get so accustomed to this diet in no time, such that you will not want to go back to your normal diet ever.

23. Never Skip Breakfast

It is believed that breakfast is known as ***break-fast*** because you literally break the night-long fast with some food in the morning. This simple myth—or fact—talks about the importance of this meal. Breakfast is definitely the most important meal of the day. There is a famous saying that goes: "Have breakfast like a king, lunch like a minister, and dinner like a pauper." This definitely shows why you should always eat a large breakfast. You can actually consume high amounts of calories during breakfast. By high, we mean high but still at a healthy level. You can eat a heavy breakfast because most of the calories gained from breakfast are lost throughout the day, and if you work out or even go for a simple walk, you will not put on weight at all.

Breakfast can include anything, but ideally, you should eat something that is not exactly heavy but is, at least, fulfilling so that your hunger will be curbed, and you will feel satiated for a long time. According to research, it is believed that you should not just eat your breakfast but you should actually eat it as soon as you wake up—specifically, within an hour of you waking up. This is supposed to enhance your metabolism and keep you motivated and active. An active and fast-working metabolism is highly essential for fast weight loss.

24. Eat This, Not That

Ghrelin is a hormone in our body that is responsible for stimulating our appetite and making us hungry. This hormone is quite important and necessary, but it can cause problems while losing weight because it will keep on making you hungry. You can suppress this hormone by doing one easy thing, which is adding around 10 to 15 grams of protein to your diet every day. You can add this protein in any way or form, but natural proteins derived from food items are always a better option. You can try adding eggs to your diet. Eggs are not only satiating, but they are also a rich source of protein, so they can actually curb your hunger.

With this, you should also try and include at least 10 grams of fiber to your diet every day. Again, this fiber can be of any kind but natural food-derived fiber is always a better option. You can also get a good amount of fiber from flaxseeds, psyllium husks, etc. Fiber is important because it satiates hunger for a long duration and can also prevent bloating, which is a common symptom of constipation. Remember to drink lots of water when you are consuming a lot of fiber.

Going low carb is an essential thing to lose weight. However, limiting all the carbs will not help you. You should try and limit carbs, such as refined carbs, which you get from muffins and bagels, and instead, you should add a small amount of good fats.

25. Measure Up!

Measuring your daily food proportions is not only a great habit while losing weight, but it is also a great thing if you want to maintain your weight. Ideally, you should not rely on simple bowls and your eyesight for measuring the portions, as these two things can betray you. Instead of relying on these things, you should buy and use good quality measuring spoons and cups. You can measure a lot of things using these cups and spoons, such as cereal, fruits, oatmeal, meal, nuts, yogurt, etc. You can also buy a small kitchen-level weighing machine, which will not only help you in measuring things for your weight loss but will also help you in baking, etc.

26. Breakfast Made Healthy

We have already covered breakfast and its importance in a previous tip. A lot of people ask how they can make a good, healthy, and fulfilling breakfast that can keep them satiated for a long time without causing any problems. You can do this in a lot of ways, and here, we highlight three really good ones. You can make and bake some healthy scones, cakes, etc., that you can consume whenever you want to have a quick yet healthy breakfast. Ideally, you should keep such things ready all the time so as to avoid a quick snack from a shop or bakery because these snacks are, more often than not, full of calories and unhealthy carbs and fats. You can also try baking the things that you normally fry or deep fry. They might not taste as good as the fried versions, but they will definitely remove a lot of calories from your diet.

While making pancakes, you should use wholegrain flour or other kinds of healthy flour. To make the pancakes healthier, you should experiment with them. You can try adding mashed, baked, or boiled sweet potatoes to the pancakes. You can also try adding blueberries, mashed spinach, and pureed greens, etc., which can increase the nutritive value of your breakfast. Quacked quinoa is also a great option.

Instead of drinking fruit juices, etc., you should try and eat the original fruits. These fruits contain fiber, which is lost when you make juices out of them. Fruits, such as grapefruit, are highly rich in fiber and should ideally be consumed all the time instead of making juice out of it.

27. Healthy Soup and Preparation of the Day

Everyone loves a hot meal. The heat makes the meal tastier and more delicious as well. However, in today's modern world, making a hot, tasty, and healthy meal every day is not always possible. You should not use these ready-to-cook meals that are packed with empty calories. Instead, to eat a hot meal every day, you can try making a huge pot full of vegetable bean soup. Then, you could divide this soup in two or more cup containers and then store them in the freezer. When you want to eat a hot meal, just take this container out of the freezer and thaw it until it gets to room temperature. Heat it over medium heat in a pot and then enjoy this delicious meal.

28. Cut the Calories

Here are some simple ways to reduce calories:

- Do not buy boxes and packs of snacks from stores. These packs more often than not contain large amounts of unhealthy ingredients that are very bad for your health. Instead of relying on these products, you should ideally buy small empty containers and then fill them with fruits and healthy snacks for you to eat at the office, school, etc.

- Although this tip might seem to be overkill, you should ideally count and label calories on each food item in your house. This will help you to keep track of your food and eating habits. It will also help you avoid over indulging and overeating. It will also become very easy for you to keep track of your diet, such that maintaining a journal will become a very easy task for you.

- Salads are very healthy, even if they are frozen. Unfortunately, the salads available outside are often very unhealthy and fattening. It is believed that salads from fast food chains are even unhealthier than the fast food options available in these chains. You should not rely on the salads available outside, and instead, you should make your own salads. You should prepare a large amount of salad on Sunday. You can then pack the salad

100 Weight Loss Tips & Stop Dieting

in five to six containers and then freeze them. You can then eat these salads every day by thawing them to room temperature.

- To make your salads even healthier, you should think of adding whole grains, corn, sprouts, etc., to them. By adding these things, you can get the best of both worlds and have a lot of nutrients together. These grains and sprouts will also help you to feel satiated and will prevent hunger for a long time. You can boil the grains and sprouts, but ideally, you should have the sprouts raw.

- If you are a sandwich lover, you should always use brown bread instead of the plain white bread. Instead of using wrap, you should use Swiss chard leaves or spinach. Cheese should be altogether skipped, or you should try to find an alternative that is healthier than regular cheese. You should add a lot of veggies to your sandwich.

- Avoid soda, soft drinks, etc., at all costs. Ideally, you should also stop consuming alcohol. Instead of consuming soda, soft drinks, iced tea, cold coffee, etc., you should add green tea, lavender tea, water, sugarless lemonade, etc., to your diet. Although these things are not that tasty, they are very healthy. Green tea is actually supposed to help you burn those calories.

- Avoid cream cheese at all costs. Instead, use peanut butter or almond butter, and spread it on your food items instead of cream cheese or simple butter. Healthy fats not only help to satiate you, but they also help curb your hunger and can even decrease your belly fats.

29. Swap It!

You can swap a lot of things in your diet that you love but are unhealthy with healthy things that taste great as well. This swapping will help you to control your hunger and will make you eat healthy stuff as well. This will also prevent you from eating unhealthy food items. You can use the following tips to learn swapping:

- Instead of eating ice cream, you should try a healthy alternative that tastes nearly the same as ice cream but is way healthier: Blend frozen bananas, peanut butter, cherries, etc., together, and then freeze this mixture. Serve this mixture as an ice cream. You can also top it with a couple of nuts.

- Instead of using spaghetti, use long juliennes of carrots, zucchini, etc. They obviously won't taste like the pasta, but they are definitely healthier.

- Instead of using fatty dips and spreads like mayonnaise, use healthy spreads like hummus, mustard, puree of roasted red pepper, and seasoned tomato puree.

- Instead of eating potato chips, try eating baked carrot chips. You can also try eating baked potato chips, but ideally, you should not eat a lot of potatoes.

- If you are making a dish that needs cream, you can try replacing it with silken tofu. You obviously cannot replace cream in all the recipes, but in some recipes, such as dairy-free chocolate mousse, it can work wonders.

- Use skimmed milk instead of full fat milk, and if you already use skimmed milk, then move over to almond milk instead.

- Instead of using white bread, always use brown bread, or use a wrap.

30. Desserts and How to Make Them Healthy

Cutting out sugar is a major part of nearly every diet in existence. Unfortunately, we love sugar, and cravings for sugar definitely are the strongest. Desserts are the most missed things on a diet. However, no need to worry; below are some of the major tips that can help you to cut out the sugar but still be able to eat desserts as well.

- Instead of dying a little daily in the memory of food and desserts, you should actually eat a small amount of sweet things every day. This will help you keep your mind calm and fresh, and you won't find yourself pining for a bowl of ice cream afterwards.

- Instead of using artificial sweeteners or sugar while making desserts, you should try adding fruits and natural sweeteners instead. You can make healthy cakes and muffins with these fruits and natural sweetener.

- You should also try adding vegetables to baked goods. These vegetables can be of any kind. You can add zucchini, carrots, sweet potatoes, etc., to your muffins and cakes. Normally, you won't be able to taste these things, and you will actually consume a lot of nutrients without even getting a taste of the veggies.

- You can also try adding natural protein powders to your desserts to make them healthier.

45

- You can replace your dessert with a bowl of healthy yogurt or low-fat and low-calorie smoothies. These will also help you remain satiated.

31. Snacks and How to make them Healthy

After desserts, snacks are definitely the most missed things when you are on a diet. However, you do not need to cut your snacks, which we have already established. Here, you will find some great tips to make your snacks healthier and your snack times better.

- It is necessary to limit your snack to around 150 calories only. You should avoid eating snacks that have more calories than this amount. You should ideally add a lot of fiber to your snacks. Some healthy snacks include fruits, seeds, etc. Remember, portions are very important.

- Instead of eating sugars, you should try to eat proteins. Proteins will not cause you to crash as they are high sources of energy. Prolonging your meal or snack is also an effective way of eating less. You can do this by consuming food that takes a lot of time to eat. For instance, you can try snacking on pods of edamame. These pods need a lot of time to eat and, thus, are a great way to prolong your meal. These pods are also high in protein and are supposed to be one of the richest protein sources. You can get around 12 grams of proteins from a single cup serving of these pods.

- Always carry your own snacks. They might seem to be a nuisance, but they can actually help you to avoid unhealthy snacks from stores, bakeries, fast-food chains, food joints, etc. Not only will this keep you on your diet, but it is also very good in keeping you from spending a lot of money on empty calories.

- Wet snacks are a better option if you are in house. Wet snacks contain a lot of water, and this will help you get full faster and will prevent bloating as well. Wet snacks commonly include melons, cherries, tomatoes, cherry tomatoes, pepper, celery, etc.

- Sprouts are also a good option for snacks. You can always eat a bowl full of sprouts to curb your hunger.

- An apple a day keeps the doctor away. Also, an apple a day will help you keep hunger at bay. Apples are full of fiber, and they have natural appetite suppressants. By eating an apple daily, you can effectively suppress your appetite.

32. Reduce the Size of Your Plate

We use dinner plates for eating our dinner, which is not a ridiculous thing at all. However, instead of using dinner plates, you should try and use salad plates for meals instead. It is believed that if you use small plates, you actually feel satiated early and do not overeat. This will definitely help you stick to your diet plan.

33. Chewing Gum All the Time

We tend to eat a lot and snack a lot if we do not have anything in our mouth. This particularly happens when a person is cooking. You can prevent this from happening if you chew gum while cooking. This will induce a sense of satiation and fulfillment.

34. Low Salt, Less Butter

Salt is infamous for causing bloating, whereas butter is famous for its high calorie content. You should avoid these two things, or use them in moderation. Try flavoring your food items, such as soups, pastas, meats, stews, etc., with stuff like onions, peppers, garlic, chili, etc. These kinds of flavorings are not only tasty, but they make food very healthy as well.

35. Go Meatless Once a Week

Although meat is very popular among people, it is also supposed to be quite unhealthy and hard to digest. It is especially not recommended when you are trying to lose weight. You should ideally adopt a meatless day, such as Meatless Monday, where you should ideally avoid meat and eat things like black beans, sweet potatoes, etc. These things are definitely healthier than meat but may not be as tasty. However, health is more important than taste, and so, you should definitely focus on health instead of taste.

36. Cut It Out

Food is not the only thing of concern when you are trying to lose weight. It is all about fooling yourself and your brain. You can do this quite effectively if you follow most of the tips given in this book. You can try and cut veggies and fruits into large chunks instead of cutting them into small pieces. Ideally, you should eat the fruit in whole form. When you have to chew a lot while eating, you get a false sense of satiation early, which can help you to reduce your food and calorie intake.

37. Think and Eat

Before taking a second serving, drink a glass of water, and then wait for a few minutes. If you still feel hungry, get that second helping; else, stop eating, and declare that you are finished.

38. Drink Your Coffee Black

If you love your regular coffee but want to lose weight, it's time to switch over to black coffee. You might think that having your regular coffee won't make much of a difference, but this kind of small switch will help in the long run. For a real coffee lover, there is no suitable replacement. So, if you can't switch over to herbal teas, at least try to take your coffee black.

Black coffee is pretty much a calorie-free beverage. When you compare the calorie count of a regular cup of black coffee or espresso to one with milk, sugar, chocolate, and other condiments, you will realize the difference it makes. One cup of espresso will only have a calorie or two in it. Sugar-laden coffee with milk can have nearly 600 calories in a single serving. All the extra flavorings and sweeteners you ask your barista to add will only pile up the calories in your diet. This means that your diet can only include coffee if you drink it completely black.

The chlorogenic acid in black coffee is said to help in speeding up weight loss. This element can help to slow down glucose production in the body, and thus, the production of fat cells is also reduced. In fact, you can also change the normal milk in your coffee to nut milk as a healthier alternative. Increasing brown fat activity can help in controlling blood sugar and blood lipid levels. The increase in calories burned will help you lose weight.

Experts have found that drinking black coffee helps in losing weight because it stimulates brown fat, which burns calories to help generate body heat. Brown fat is different from the other fat that is in your body. It burns sugar and fat to produce body heat when it is cold.

Coffee beans contain various biologically active substances that can affect your metabolism. Other than caffeine, it has theobromine and theophylline as well. Black coffee also has antioxidants that will boost your weight loss process. The caffeine will be effective in increasing metabolic activity and boosting energy levels. Many people drink coffee as a stimulant before they exercise every day. Caffeine blocks adenosine and increases the release of dopamine and norepinephrine. this will help you feel awake and energized. The caffeine from your black coffee will also help to reduce untimely food cravings and help your body burn fat with more efficiency. So, you can now enjoy your coffee without worrying about your weight.

39. Eat Your Dinner Early

Eating your dinner earlier is another great tip to help you control your weight. The modern-day lifestyle is quite unhealthy in many ways. We eat untimely meals or just skip them altogether. Eating a late dinner is a common habit among people who tend to be overweight. Some studies show that eating all your regular meals earlier in the day can help in boosting weight loss and suppressing hunger pangs. So, you have to start considering the fact that it is not just about what you eat but also about when you eat. Instead of having dinner at 10 p.m. or right before bed, you should consider fixing dinner time to around 7 p.m.

Trust us when we say that it can make a lot of difference. The last meal of your day should be early and light, and there are many reasons for it. Scheduling your meal timings helps in conditioning your internal rhythm. This rhythm of your body helps it adjust to changes in sleep, eating, digestion, etc. Your meal timings will thus have an effect on the regulation of your body weight, metabolism, and various other health factors.

When you eat your dinner earlier, it increases the duration of your overnight fast. The time between dinner and breakfast allows your body to burn extra fat. Fasting initiates a process called ketosis that helps the body burn stored fat. This means that you will be losing weight while you sleep if you just eat early. Early dinners are much better for your digestive system, and having healthy digestion will aid in weight loss. The later you eat your dinner, the more likely it is that the food will just lie in your intestines or get stored as fat instead of being used.

Eating late also increases the risk of indigestion and heartburn. This will indirectly affect the quality of your sleep. Avoid eating any midnight snack if you want a healthy circadian rhythm or are trying to lose weight. Eating at least a few hours before sleeping will allow the food to be digested, and you can sleep better in a sated state. A late dinner can also cause bloating and water retention in the body. However, you also have to maintain a healthy time gap between dinner and bedtime.

If you eat early but sleep too late, it will just cause other problems and make it easier for you to reach for unhealthy snacks. Start your day early with breakfast, and fix a meal schedule for the whole day. Go to bed within two to three hours of dinner. This will let your body adjust in a healthy way. Thus, you won't have to skip meals and starve yourself to lose weight. Just eat better food and earlier.

40. Be Patient

While you embark on this weight loss journey, patience is of utmost importance. You cannot and should not try to lose a lot of weight in a short amount of time. This is not going to help your body and will instead cause more harm. When you follow fad diets or starve yourself to lose weight, it is more likely that you will soon be gaining it all back again. You may even see the numbers on the scale go down if you don't eat for a couple of days, but that is not real weight loss. Most people embark on their weight loss journey to try and see amazing results in as little time as possible. A lot of people lack patience and give up on healthy eating or exercise when they don't see quick results.

When you are on a diet and establishing a new eating pattern for yourself, it is natural to experience some ups and downs. You will need to be patient while you are experiencing these highs and lows. There might be days when you go off the diet plan and eat things that are not really healthy for you. You need to be patient with yourself and not feel guilty about being unable to be as disciplined as you aim to be. You can always go back on a diet the next day. However, if you are impatient and let small slip-ups demotivate you, it will be harder to get back on track. You have to be forgiving and patient with yourself if you want to establish a healthy pattern and achieve long-term weight loss.

All the diet tips given in this book will work effectively and surely. However, there is no guarantee that they will give you the instantly gratifying results that you may be looking for. You won't lose 10 pounds in five days or fit into your skinny jeans in two weeks. The process will take time but will effectively help you lose and manage your weight if you remain persistent and patient. Being impatient will just cause you to get off track and have to start all over again.

Instead, you can utilize the dietary tips given here and allow yourself to make a healthy lifestyle change for better long-term results. You have to be patient and aim for sustained weight loss. Don't start binging on junk food just because the numbers on your scale don't show significant change in a month. Weight loss is not just about the numbers and quick changes in body shape. The healthy dietary changes will slowly but surely facilitate long-term weight loss and help you get fit and healthy again.

Nicholas Bjorn

Chapter 3 – 20 Exercise Tips to Lose Weight

Dieting is just one part of the game or one side of the coin in weight loss. If you genuinely want to lose weight, mere dieting won't suffice and is not recommended at all. Instead, you should ideally add a regular workout plan to your routine.

Pairing good diet habits with regular workouts will help you lose weight more effectively. Some people find different excuses to avoid working out, but this activity is essential if you want to lose weight. You do not need to do any specific kind of workout; any kind of exercise is okay if you it helps you lose weight.

1. Commit to a Set Amount of Time

While many people commit to working out as their new year's resolution, few follow through. This is because of the lack of commitment and discipline. They don't really put in much thought or effort into when they're actually going to work out. If you want to lose weight, you have to be ready to commit to a set day and time for exercise. You also have to consider how long you will work out. It could be anything from 20 minutes to an hour; it is up to you. However, you have to stick to this timing and not stop before the timer runs out. If you have dedicated yourself to a 30-minute workout, stick to it. It may seem a little hard in the beginning, but if you push yourself, it gets easier. Soon, you will easily be able to increase the duration of your workout well beyond what you had initially planned on. Committing to your days and durations for workouts will actively help you lose a lot of weight. Diet and exercise will go hand in hand when it comes to weight loss. You cannot skip your workouts and expect the results you want to see.

2. Build a Workout Routine

Building a workout routine is important for weight loss as well. First, only doing cardio will not help you much. Cardio should definitely be a part of your workout but not the only exercise you do. When you are aiming for weight loss, you have to think about what kind of workout you should be doing. Planning a workout routine before you start will help you see better results and guide you along the way. Don't go overboard with cardio, and make sure you include at least some weight training. Weight training helps boost metabolism for a longer period than cardio does. So, mix the two, and create a routine for yourself. You can have three days of cardio with two days of strength training every week to start with. The days and duration of your workout will depend on you and your needs. Remember not to overdo it, and allow yourself recovery days. Similarly, you can switch up between different types of exercise on different days of the week according to your preference. Instead of going to the gym every day, you can even add a day or two or some sport that you like, such as tennis or swimming. Otherwise, fix your workout routine according to the different areas of the body that you want to focus on. On Mondays and Wednesdays, you can focus on the abs, while Tuesdays and Thursdays could be leg days. You get the drift. Just build on your personal workout routine. You can keep changing it along the way to see what works best. This will help you lose weight in the best way possible and see real results from your exercise.

Use these tips to build your workout routine:

- First, determine your situation. Are you just trying to lose weight, or do you want to build muscle and bulk up? Write down what your goals are so that you have a clear idea of what you want to accomplish from the workout. Then, think about how much time you can devote to working out. Dedicating 45 minutes to one hour a day would be ideal, but it isn't always possible for everyone. However, you have to take some time to figure out what your possible workout duration is. You can develop the most efficient workout routine according to your workout duration. What you can accomplish in one hour can also be done in 30 minutes if you exercise the right way. Strength training can burn twice the calories that cardio does within half the time. You also need to figure out where you are planning to work out. It could be at home, at the gym, or even at a park. The place where you work out will help you determine the kind of training you can do. This is because you don't have the same equipment that a gym has if you exercise at home. Your workout has to be adjusted according to the tools you have at hand.

- The next step is to figure out what kind of exercises you should be doing. The best workout will be the one that you know you can actually stick with. Don't choose something that seems too difficult for you because it will set you up for failure. You don't need to make your workout routine too complicated. It should just be efficient and simple while helping you improve your body. To begin with, you should figure out a full body routine and do this at least three times a week. Ideally, you should try working out five days the week. Your routine should include exercises that work on every part of your body. There are specific moves designed for the quads and others for the butt and hamstrings. Quad exercises include squats, box jumps, and lunges. The hamstrings and butt will improve with deadlifts, step-ups, and hip raises. You will also need to do exercises for the push muscles that include your shoulders, chest, and triceps. These include bench press, push-ups, dips, and overhead press. Exercises for the pull muscles will focus on the back, grip, and biceps. This will include bent-over rows, pull-ups, and chin-ups. Dedicate some exercise for your core, which includes the abdomen and lower back. These exercises will include planks, mountain climbers, side planks, jumping knee tucks, and hanging leg raise. You can ask an instructor or just watch videos online to learn how to do all these exercises in the correct way. You can choose one exercise for each target area, and that will make up your workout routine for the week. You can switch up the exercises every other week to keep it fun. Focus on these basic exercises first, and get stronger. Then, you can move on to more complicated exercises to help you burn more calories. If you do compound movements that work on multiple muscles at once, you will only have to do a few exercises in your routine. Compound movements will make your workouts more efficient.

- You have to figure out how many sets and reps you should do. A set involves repetitions of an exercise without stopping. So, doing 10 crunches will mean one set of ten reps. Typically, you should first do a warm-up and then move on to the sets and reps. Try doing three to five sets for each exercise in a single workout. The reps per set can be seven to eight when you are first beginning. If you want to burn fat and build muscle at the same time, you should try at least 10 to 15 repetitions per set. If 15 reps are easy for you, increase the difficulty of that movement or increase the weights. When you do 1 to 5 reps, it helps in building strength and dense muscle. If you do 6 to 12 reps, you will be building muscle strength and muscle size. Doing more than 12 reps will allow you to build muscle endurance. Don't stress too much about how many sets and reps you should do. To begin with, try lighter weights and more reps, and you can build from there. Just focus on getting stronger with each workout you do. These workouts should push you and help you burn as many calories as possible. If you don't strain yourself a little, you won't lose weight, even if you exercise for an hour.

- You need to keep track of how long you should wait between each set. The time can be adjusted according to how healthy the individual is. You need a small break between each set to rest, but the break should not be too long, just as much as necessary. If you are doing heavy lifting reps within the 1 to 3 range, rest for about 3 to 5 minutes. If you are doing 4 to 7 reps of strength lifting, rest for 2 to 3 minutes between each set. If you are doing 8 to 12 reps for size or strength, rest for a minute or two. If you are doing more than 13 reps to build endurance, just rest long enough to help you recover before the next set. You should just focus on doing the best that you can. So, your rest period between sets does not have to be a specific time that everyone else follows. It should just be enough to allow you to recover and repeat.

- You have to find the right weight that you should be lifting. Don't shy away from weights, even if you don't want to build a muscular body. Weights will help build strength, tone, and muscle. The more muscle you build, the more fat you will burn. Trial and error will allow you to determine how much weight you should lift. You have to lift enough to be able to get through your whole set, but not so much that you cannot do any more exercises after the set. It has to be between too heavy and too light. You can work with your body weight, but then you have to make your exercises a little more difficult over time. When 20 push-ups become easy for you, increase it to 25 to 30, and so on.

- How long should your workout be? Generally, 45 minutes of a workout routine is efficient in helping anyone burn their excess weight. If you do around 3 to 5 sets of 5 different exercises, you will find 45 minutes more than enough. However, you also have to figure in some time for warming up before the workout and stretching after you are done. If you increase the intensity of your workout, you can decrease the duration of it. A highly intense workout in lesser time will give you better results than if you did the opposite.

- How many days in a week should you train? Some people might tell you to exercise every single day of the week. However, we will tell you differently. Firstly, you may not have the time to do this. Secondly, you probably don't want to. You have to build a workout routine that you can continue for a long time. You cannot be training seven days a week unless you are a professional athlete. So, try at least three to five workouts every week. You get time to rest and pick yourself back up again if you follow this routine. Just try exercising every alternate day if you can't do it continuously. Otherwise, work out on weekdays and enjoy the weekend to rest. Just remember to exercise and stay active if you are serious about losing weight.

- Lastly, keep track of everything. Write down details about when you work out, what exercises you did, and how your weight is changing. It will help you maintain and adjust your workout in the long term.

Here is an example of a workout routine if you want to lose weight:

- Cardio twice a week. Each session should be at least 40 to 50 minutes.

- Strength training twice a week. Each session should be an hour.

- High-intensity interval training once a week. The session can be of 20 minutes.

- Keep two days of the week for active recovery.

It doesn't necessarily have to be this particular plan. It just has to be a routine similar to this that really helps you get active and burn the fat. Following a routine will help you strain your body in a healthy way consistently and thus lose weight. It's not a big deal if you miss a workout once in a while. However, you should definitely get back on track the next day.

3. Set a Schedule for Your Workouts

If you are serious about a regular workout, schedule a fixed time for it. Don't just try to fit your workout in here and there. This will only give you more opportunities to back out of it whenever you can grab the chance. When you make it a fixed part of your routine, it will grow into a lifelong healthy habit that you will thank yourself for in the long run. Make your workout a predictable task in your day. This will let you know that this particular time of the day is specifically assigned only for exercise. You cannot make excuses about being too busy the whole day to find time to exercise. So how do you commit time for a workout? Well, when you are just starting out, you have to try to work out at least 3 to 4 days a week. Fix those particular days in the week when you can make time to exercise. Next, figure out what time works best for you, and schedule your workout well in advance for those timings on those days. Plan it out well, and note it down on your phone calendar or just a note on the fridge. Don't budge from the plan.

4. Try High-intensity Interval Workouts

High-intensity interval training or HIIT is a workout that includes intense activity for a short period of time, followed by a low-intensity activity. HIIT is very convenient for people who usually have busy schedules. HIIT workouts can be as short as 4 to 7 minutes and are very versatile. Studies show that HIIT workouts tend to burn more calories and fat even if done only for a short period of time. The workout can also cause your body to be in hyper drive, because of which you burn calories as much as 24 hours after your workout. You can incorporate HIIT into your workout regimen. For example, you can run as fast as you can for 40 seconds, then rest for 20 seconds. You can also do bodyweight exercises for a determined amount of time and then rest afterwards. Moreover, there is a Tabata training method through which you can complete a workout in just 4 minutes.

5. Power Up Your Run

Running is probably the best cardio exercise there is. It helps in improving cardiovascular health and boosts blood circulation. Running can build the foundation for any other fitness activity. It's not just for losing weight. When you add strength training to your running, it is the best combination to lose weight and improve overall health. This is why you should consider powering up your runs. Don't just run continuously for 45 minutes on the treadmill. Instead, add exercises like squats and lunges in between the run itself. It will push your body to the next level and boost the fat burning process in a major way. You can start your warm-up and then do around 15 minutes of a moderately paced run. Then, add some burpees, lunges, squats, push-ups, or pull-ups in between. You can do all of these exercises between two running periods. You can also keep running and stop every couple of minutes from doing at least 30 seconds of any of these exercises. You need to endure at least 30 minutes of this kind of workout if you want to really boost your metabolism and burn more fat. Take time to cool down after this kind of workout. Run at a slower pace as you finish your power workout.

6. Switch It Up

Your body can quickly adapt to your fitness plan, so it is a good idea to switch up your cardio and strength training every now and then. The change doesn't have to be dramatic. You can increase the intensity or the duration of your workout. You can also try other fitness activities. Discovering a new sport or training method can be both fun and exciting. Try dancing classes, yoga, Pilates, Zumba, CrossFit, or any sport. If you are lifting weights, you should also gradually increase the weights to continue reaping benefits from the exercise. The main idea is to keep challenging your body to avoid a weight loss plateau.

7. Use High-quality Clothes While Working Out

It is important to wear the right workout clothes to keep you safe and comfortable throughout your workout. Wearing proper running shoes while jogging can prevent injuries and can also help you maintain your balance. It is difficult to stay focused on your workout if you are not comfortable. Choose clothes that are right for your body and offer flexibility so that you can move freely. Choose fabrics that have moisture-wicking properties. These types of fabric keep your skin dry and your body cool while you exercise. Women should also invest in a sports bra that provides adequate support.

8. Find a Workout Partner

Having a partner or buddy can motivate you to work out even when you are feeling lazy. Knowing that there is someone waiting for you can enable you to push your excuses aside and meet your fitness goals. Make sure that you find someone who can inspire you to do better.

Your spouse can be great workout partner as well. They are competitive but not crazy about it. You can even make this a romantic activity.

9. Choose Your Tunes

Workouts can be boring without music. Search for music that can get you in the mood to work out. There are several athletes who opt to listen to relaxing music while doing hard workouts, whereas there are those who opt for upbeat music. Choose music that can motivate you to do better in your workout. As a cautionary note, make sure that you are not playing your music too loud, especially when you are working out outdoors, so you can still hear cars and warning sounds.

There are many CDs and albums available in the market solely made for the purpose of exercise. You can find some soulful and classic Indian music for Yoga and some peppy music for aerobics in one CD. Check out the market, or browse online stores.

10. Pay Attention to Your Form

Make sure that you maintain proper form throughout your workout. Getting injured because of improper form while working out can only prevent you from achieving your weight loss goal. Enlisting the help of a fitness trainer for the first month can help you achieve proper form. You should also remember that you should never sacrifice your form to complete more repetitions or to lift heavier weights.

Exercise-related injuries are extremely common and painful as well. These injuries can be simple things, such as pulling a muscle, but can also be something horrifying like muscle or ligament tear, fracture, etc.

11. Do Compound Exercises

You can maximize your workout time by doing compound movements instead of isolated exercise. Isolated exercises like bicep curls can only work a particular muscle, whereas compound exercises can target multiple muscle groups at once. This means that you will get the benefit of a full-body exercise with just a few exercises. Compound movements are also beneficial for strengthening your body. Examples of compound exercises include lunges, squats, pull-ups, shoulder press, and bench press.

Some compound forms of exercises include dancing, dance aerobics, etc. These forms are highly effective and useful in losing weight in a very healthy manner.

12. Use the Body that You Have

Exercising in a gym that has various machines and equipment has its own advantages, but do not think that you cannot have a great workout without fancy equipment. There are many people who manage to exercise and lose weight through bodyweight training. Bodyweight exercises are movements that use your own body as a form of weight and resistance. These exercises include push-ups, burpees, and air squats. Bodyweight exercise is also recommended for people who don't have the time or budget to go to a gym.

It is a well-known myth that you need to be rich to gain weight and to lose it as well. It is also believed that you need to eat a lot of fancy stuff to lose weight and to gain muscles. If this were the case, then prisoners living in prisons would not look so buff and muscular. Instead, they would look weak, frail, and skinny. This sole fact debunks this popular myth.

13. Accept Discomfort

If you are overweight and unused to any exercise, you have to expect some discomfort. Don't assume that it will be easy. If you truly want to get fit, accept the initial discomfort as part of the package. Discomfort is not the same as pain. If you are in real pain or hurt yourself, you need to stop immediately, and seek medical attention. However, if you just stop your workout because you feel tired, it is not the same. This is why we emphasize the importance of fixing the duration for your workout as well. You cannot do 10 minutes of a run and give up. It will be tiring and tough initially, but you will get past that stage soon. You need to commit yourself to at least a month of a fixed workout routine. This whole month might seem long and tiring for you, but it will soon become a habit. You might experience some cramps and soreness when you exercise for the first week or so, but it is to be expected. You are pushing your body out of its usual comfort zone and changing your unhealthy routine to a better one. You have to know the difference between good "pain" and bad pain. If the first signs of discomfort make you stop exercising, you will barely ever exercise at all. The more effort you start putting into your workout, and the more you push yourself to a new level, the more discomfort you will initially feel. However, this passes, and you will soon be able to go through entire workouts without a break. The real pain is when you are injured or hurt yourself in some way while exercising. This is the only time you can excuse yourself out of a workout without guilt. Otherwise, learn to accept the discomfort, and look forward to the results and the achievement of your weight loss goals.

It is important that you know you will be sore from increasing activity, but it's crucial you know the difference between discomfort and pain.

14. Try Something New

So, exercise is obviously a crucial part of losing weight. However, exercise does not only mean going to the gym and doing strenuous workouts. There are many other ways in which you can exercise your body and even have fun while doing it. Why don't you try something new? This will motivate you and make you look forward to this form of exercise. Does the idea of rock climbing excite you? Well, this is also a form of exercise and would be a great way to lose weight.

Sign up for some rock climbing classes or sessions. If you like running, then don't just stick to the treadmill. Go out for a run around the park or new neighborhoods. This can be a refreshing change. Even better, you can sign up for a marathon. It will give you a goal to look forward to. Train for your marathon until the day comes, and you will reap the satisfaction of completing it. Meanwhile, you will also be losing a lot of weight. Trying something new will motivate you to stick to your exercise schedule, even if you are bored with your usual workouts. You can even try some Pilates or Zumba sessions to switch things up. Working out does not have to be as boring as you expect it to be. A lot of these activities won't even feel like exercise, but you will be enjoying while reaping the benefits of burning a lot of calories.

The following are some great new ways to exercise while having fun:

- Hiking: Just put your hiking shoes on, and get out of your house. Explore different hiking trails near you. Get a hiking buddy, or join a group. There are many great hiking spots that you can explore, and you will be burning fat the whole time that you go on this adventure. Hiking is a great weekend workout activity to look forward to.

- Rock climbing: Rock climbing is a little more intense than some other activities. You have to be fit and be careful while you do it. This form of exercise is great for the arm, back, and forearms in particular. You can check what your level is, and go on the climbing route that is suitable for you. You can also go to a nearby center that teaches you rock climbing in artificial setups.

- Dancing: Dancing is one of the most fun ways to burn fat. Sign up for dancing classes, or just blast some music and dance by yourself. Swing dancing and hip-hop will get you drenched in sweat in no time. You can try Zumba or the Tango as well. There are so many different types of dancing classes you can sign up for; just choose something that catches your fancy. You will be learning something new, meeting new people, and losing a lot of weight along the way. Dancing will make you feel good mentally and physically.

- Martial arts: If you are an avid movie buff, you have probably been interested in martial arts at some point or the other. Use this opportunity to sign up and learn it now. You will burn calories and also learn self-defense. It will also make you feel like a real badass.

- Clean: Yes, cleaning is also a form of exercise. Nobody likes cleaning up their house or room, but it really gets you moving. So, play some music, and clean every inch of your room. It'll keep you active and also help you get something done. There's nothing better than coming home to a clean house. While you clean your house, you are also keeping your body fit.

- Yoga: Yoga helps in increasing flexibility and building strength, and it also helps you relax on another level.

There are so many types of yoga you can try out, and it really works. While you will be burning fat, you will also improve your mental wellbeing.

Just try out any new activity that will get you up and about.

15. Don't Forget to Rest

Your desire to lose weight might just be too much that it pushes you over your limit. Make sure that you give your body enough time to recover. Do not work the same set of muscle groups in consecutive days. While it is important to challenge your body, it is also crucial that you do not push yourself to the point of fatigue and exhaustion. This can have a detrimental effect on your body and morale.

Sleeping is a very effective form of rest, but it can be a nuisance if you lead a busy life. Instead, try doing various breathing exercises and meditations that will help you to relax yourself and will help you to keep yourself active and well rested. Power naps should be incorporated in your day-to-day life as well.

16. Realize that You Can't Do it Alone

It pays to invest in a trainer if you are new to working out. A trainer can correct your form and observe your progress. Make sure that you find a trainer who has your best interest in mind. You can inquire about the trainer's experience and speak with his or her regular clients to understand his or her methods.

You can also ask for the help of like-minded people. There are a lot of people who are passionate about fitness and living a healthy lifestyle. You can join support groups that can provide you with more information on how you can achieve your own weight loss goals. Hiring a gym teacher is a great option as well, but it is costly. Ideally, a good friend who is fit or wants to get in better shape will be your best option. This kind of friend will keep you motivated, and the competition that arises from this kind of friendship will be a great motivator as well.

17. New Rewards

Have you reached any of your goals? If so, you should allow yourself to feel proud and pleased with yourself. You should also reward yourself. Build the habit of rewarding yourself each time you reach a new goal. This will go a long way in keeping you focused and motivated to keep improving.

Instead of indulging on fast food, snacks, or ice cream, treat yourself to some new gym gear. There are many really stylish brands you can choose from when you are looking at workout clothing. Spend some cash on a new outfit or gym shoes, and avoid the guilt that some rewards can cause. Maybe you have always wanted to start a home gym. Look into some equipment for your home. Buy a set of dumb bells, and use them at home.

Whatever you decide, the main thing is to change your attitude toward how you reward yourself. Rewards do not have to be unhealthy or bad for you. Change your attitude, as well as your body, so think healthy and stay healthy.

18. Track Your Body

Another rewarding way to keep track of your weight loss journey is to track the changes in your body and use pictures. A picture is said to be worth a thousand words, and this definitely holds true. When you're on a weight loss journey, seeing the changes with your own eyes will be much better than anyone else pushing you on. This will motivate you, even more, to keep going. When you see real results from all your effort, you will be more likely to keep going. You might not see drastic changes in a short period of time, but they will definitely happen slowly.

Most people are motivated to start on their weight loss journey in the first place because they want to improve their body image. They either want to look a certain way or fit into certain clothes. So, tracking the changes will not only motivate you but also help you notice if you are slacking. If you don't see any real changes, you will also know that you are doing something wrong. It will give you a chance to assess your workout routine and your diet as well. Nonetheless, the main purpose of tracking progress is to motivate you.

Take measurements of your body, and note them down in a diary according to date. However, don't keep taking measurements too frequently. It is impractical to expect to go from a size 10 to a size 8 in 5 days. Instead, measure yourself every 2 to 3 weeks. This will be a much more realistic method and also be more likely to show you changes.

Also, take pictures. Taking before and after pictures during a weight loss journey can be immensely motivating and gratifying. Take one picture of the same clothes and in the same poses once a week. Over the next few months, you can compare these pictures side by side and notice the difference. Don't aim for quick perfection, and instead, look forward to healthy improvement over time. Don't set a goal like becoming a size zero in 2 months. You can be a bigger size and still be healthy and fit. Use the measurement tracking and pictures to help you keep going on your efforts for weight loss. Even the slightest changes can be very important for your mental strength. Studies have shown that people who tried this particular tip were more likely to keep eating right and exercising than those who didn't.

Another study conducted at Columbia University showed that people who were trying to lose weight while being motivated by body image were more likely to succeed while they used this kind of tracking. So, it is not just about checking the number on your weighing scale because numbers can be deceiving. When you see pictures of yourself and how your clothes fit differently, you can definitely feel the changes in body weight yourself. Your pictures will always be a great reminder for you to see how far you have come with persistence, effort, and patience.

19. Watch Your Clothes

Clothes play a very important role in a weight loss regimen. As said earlier, try to use clothes that are highly comfortable and can absorb sweat.

You should also prevent and avoid baggy clothes and instead wear form-fitting clothes. Form-fitting clothes always remind you that you are supposed to be losing weight, and they do not let you forget about your regimen. Baggy clothes hide your body and, more often than not, this can lead to forgetfulness about your diet and exercise regimen. So, even when you are relaxing in your house, you should definitely wear form-fitting clothes that will keep you on track all the time.

20. Patience

Regular exercise is an important aspect of losing weight permanently. As we have mentioned earlier in the book, patience is of utmost importance in your weight loss journey. You have to exercise this patience even when it comes to working out. Be patient, and follow through with your workouts. Be patient as you wait for the results to show. Don't expect your workout to be very easy or for it to show you instant results. You are not going to lose 5 pounds in a couple of days, no matter how strenuous your workout regimen is. Your goal may be to build more muscle or to increase your flexibility. You could be aiming to lose overall weight or just in some areas. No matter what the goal is, you will have to be persistent and patient. You will reach your goal weight at some point, but you cannot be impatient about it. You will not see any changes happen overnight. However, if you establish a practical regimen of exercise that you are able to follow on a daily basis, you will be able to see results in the long term. It will be gradual, and you will have to put in day-to-day efforts. That is the only way you can see improvement. Patience and consistency are important. You may train extremely hard for weeks and then you may just give up one day. However, you have to keep exercising if you want your results to remain.

Don't stop exercising if you are unhappy with your initial results. Don't stop exercising if your waist measurement hasn't changed after 10 days. Don't stop exercising if you look the same as you did a month before you started working out. It takes different amounts of time for different people, and the results will vary as well. Don't get impatient if your workout buddy loses more weight than you did even if you started out together. Their body is completely different from yours, and you should just use this as motivation to keep going and aim for similar results. Do not expect instant results if you want long-term benefits from your exercise and dietary changes. Be patient, and see how your efforts pay off.

Nicholas Bjorn

Chapter 4 – 20 Lifestyle Tips for Weight Loss

Deciding to lose weight can affect your entire life. There are countless fad diets and programs that promise quick fixes but do not offer real results. In fact, if you try to lose weight by doing fad diets, you can actually ruin your body and can cause many problems to your health. Moreover, the weight lost due to fad diets is not permanent, but the health problems arising due to these diets definitely are.

You cannot simply lose weight by dieting or just exercising. You need a lot of planning and also need to understand your body. To lose weight successfully, you should evaluate your lifestyle and change your negative and unhealthy habits. You need to drop those unhealthy foods and replace them with healthy albeit tasty stuff. You also need to work hard to drop those extra calories.

1. Change Your Mindset

Going through the process of losing weight can make you stronger and more confident. It will also help you realize some aspects of yourself. You will learn the kind of physical activities you enjoy and what healthy foods you like. Most importantly, you would understand the importance of maintaining a healthy weight. Your reasons for losing weight should go beyond wanting to "look good." You should also expect to feel better, more energized, and healthier after losing weight.

Remember, losing weight is not a physical thing; it is a state of mind. You cannot lose weight simply by concentrating only on the physical aspect. Similarly, weight loss not only affects your body but concerns your mind as well. You feel active, fresh, and happy.

2. Make It a Commitment, and Write It Down

Permanent weight loss takes time and effort. Once you decide to start eating right and working out, you should make it a life-long commitment. You should be ready to make permanent changes in your lifestyle. Write your goals down in your journal. Whenever you feel like you are losing motivation, read what you have written to remind yourself of your commitment.

Remember, commitment is the most important thing. As long as you are committed to your goal, you will stay put and concentrate on losing weight. As said earlier, read your journal to keep yourself on track. You can also try downloading an app to keep yourself committed.

3. Document Your Weight Loss

Documenting your weight loss can keep you motivated. You can keep a journal to record your thoughts. You can also take photographs of yourself before and after weight loss to help keep yourself motivated to continue with achieving your goal. Seeing how far you have come would also give you a sense of accomplishment.

Documenting your weight loss is not only a fun way to keep you motivated, but it is also a way to keep your habits and routine in check. Looking at your progress every day, even if it is just a little progress, will keep you motivated. You can achieve better results if you keep an eye on your progress. With this, you should ideally write everything down, including your measurements, your weight loss, your weight gain, your muscle gain, your BMI, calories, etc.

4. Morning Routine

If you want to lose weight, you need to start your day the right way. Your morning routine sets the tone for the rest of your day. There are a few things that you can start doing each morning to stimulate weight loss in your body. Everyone knows that waking up early and being a morning person is a healthy lifestyle habit. Studies show that those people who wake up earlier in the morning tend to be happier, healthier, and more successful. So, the next time that anyone advises you to wake up at dawn, you should really consider it, but for now, let's focus on the benefits of waking up early if you want to lose weight.

The following are some habits that should be a part of your morning routine if you want your weight loss journey to be more successful:

- Wake up as early as you can, and give yourself some time before you need to head out to work. Don't wake up 5 minutes before you need to rush out. This will prevent you from carrying out a healthy morning routine for yourself. Sleep earlier at night so that you get adequate sleep and feel well-rested in the morning. If you don't sleep well, skip breakfast, and go through the whole day tired, you are less likely to be a fit person.

- Drink some warm water as soon as you wake up. Drinking a tall glass of water will kickstart your body in the morning. Squeeze some lemon juice into the water for an added boost. This trick is considered helpful in burning belly fat. You can also try having a spoon of apple cider vinegar with water for the same reason. Staying hydrated the whole day will help you lose more weight. People often mistake their thirst for water for hunger and eat more when they drink less water. Drinking a glass of water before a meal will also prevent you from overeating because it gives you the sensation of feeling full. Water is actually a natural appetite suppressant that will work to your benefit. It is also helpful in enhancing your metabolism, and you will burn more calories. Starting your day by drinking a tall glass of water and staying hydrated will allow your body to remove toxins and wastes easily.

- Give yourself time to have a proper high-protein breakfast. Having a healthy meal in the morning will keep you fueled all day. It is also an important factor in preventing unhealthy food cravings between your main meals. Many people skip breakfast because they don't have time or just because they think it'll help them lose weight. However, it does the exact opposite. People who eat a regular breakfast tend to be fitter than someone who skips breakfast. However, you also have to consider what you eat. Your breakfast should be high in protein if you are aiming for weight loss. This means that you should eat more eggs, Greek yogurt, tofu, etc. Protein will help to reduce the level of ghrelin in the body. Ghrelin is also called the hunger hormone. Avoid eating sugary foods, such as cereals or any junk food. These will only add calories and increase your weight. If you eat the right foods in the morning, it will give you more energy and also aid in burning fat.

- Drink a cup of herbal tea or black coffee. The antioxidants and the caffeine will be helpful in giving you an added boost. It will also help you focus more in the morning and stimulate you to go through a morning workout.

- Try working out in the morning hours instead of the evening. Mornings are the best time in the day to get a workout in. Research shows that people who exercise in the morning will tend to consume fewer calories throughout the day. A morning workout is more effective in burning fat and extra weight around the abdominal area as compared to working out at any other time of the day. Set aside time in the morning to exercise in any form you like. It could be a run, a HIIT workout, or just a swim. Any of it will stimulate weight loss, reduce appetite, and help you burn more calories.

- Try to get some exposure to sunlight in the morning. You could just sit outside with your coffee for a few minutes or workout under the sun. Certain studies say that getting adequate exposure to sunlight in the day also plays a role in weight loss and overall health. An added bonus is that you will be getting some important vitamin D as well.

- Weigh yourself in the mornings. This is the time of the day that you should note down your weight. Don't be scared of the weighing scale, and don't judge yourself on the basis of the numbers. It will just give you an idea of your body weight and help you measure progress. Seeing the numbers reduce in the morning will also motivate you to keep working toward weight loss. It will also help you make any appropriate adjustments to your diet or workout routine. If you have gained weight, you need to exercise a little more and have better control over what or how much you eat. If the numbers are reducing, you are probably doing it right. This is why regular weighing can be a good idea in the morning.

- Set intentions for the rest of your day. Plan out what you are going to do on that day. Don't go through your day without any direction. It will prevent you from being as productive as you could otherwise be. Practicing mindfulness in the morning is also considered helpful for your physical and mental wellbeing. It will relieve stress and boost your focus. It will also help you in losing weight because you will have better control over your emotions and thoughts. You will be less likely to binge on junk food or do any emotional eating. Just take five minutes to be mindful every morning, and see the difference it makes.

Start implementing any of the above in your morning routine, and begin your day the right way.

5. Predefined Hours

Set a schedule for yourself. This can be an extremely useful tool throughout your life. You can define the hours you spend on all your tasks throughout the day. Set aside time on the previous night or in the morning, and make a schedule for yourself. Note down what task you will be doing at any particular time of the day. Don't drift through the day without any direction. Everyone could use the help of a schedule. Make sure you assign a particular time for all your meals and workout during that day. Don't try to squeeze it in between work. Your health is much more important than work. You will also be able to be more productive and successful if you eat well and take care of your body. So, when the clock strikes at 1 p.m., make sure you are eating your lunch. If you have set your workout time for 9 a.m., don't allow yourself to do anything else at that time. Similarly, you can focus solely on work on your predefined hours for work.

Moreover, set a bedtime for yourself, even if it may seem juvenile to you. As we have mentioned earlier in the book, your body has a circadian rhythm that plays an important role. Setting a bedtime for every day will help your body function better. It will also help you lose more weight in the long run because of this fixed routine. So, take out time to define hours for all your tasks. It will work in your favor.

6. Find Your Motivation

Everyone has their own reason to lose weight. Make a list of the reasons why you want to lose weight to remind yourself to pursue your goal. For added motivation, you can also find motivational quotes that you can relate to.

You can also get motivated by reading or listening to successful weight loss stories. You will realize that everyone faces challenges while losing weight. You might even pick up some tips from people who have already successfully lost weight and maintained a healthy weight. If you do not know any such person in real life, the internet can always help you. There are many forums and websites online, dedicated solely to weight loss techniques and methods. You can find lots of people who have completed their journey of weigh loss or currently on their road to lose weight. You can also share your own journey on such platforms and thus gain a lot of support and motivation.

 A lot of people have different ways to keep them motivated. Some people love to dance while some people love to have a chat with a loved one. Some people also like to read motivational books, both fiction and nonfiction. Some people also like to sing or listen to music to motivate themselves. Choose your own way. If you have a hobby, such as gardening, etc., you should take it up and have fun doing it. This fun portion will refresh your mind and will make you more active and dedicated to achieving your goals.

7. Plan a SMART Goal

Simply wanting to lose weight is not enough. You should also set a SMART goal to achieve it. SMART stands for specific, measurable, achievable, relevant, and time-bound.

A specific goal is much easier to accomplish than a broad one. Keep it measurable by tracking your progress regularly. This way, you will know whether you are on the right track. Achievable goals mean that they are not too extreme. You shouldn't expect yourself to change overnight. Have the patience to achieve your goal gradually. Relevant goals mean that they are important to you. Remind yourself constantly of why you want to lose weight in the first place. Time-bound means that you have to set a reasonable deadline to achieve your goal. This establishes a sense of urgency and prevents your goal from being overtaken by your daily activities.

If you decide to start eating more vegetables, then you should determine a way to start incorporating them into your diet. If you want to work out, then you should set a time and place to do it. It is also equally important to follow through with whatever strategy you decide on.

Do not set unrealistic goals and then try to achieve them. More often than not, these unrealistic goals are impossible to achieve and, thus, can actually break your confidence and dedication. It is a good thing to have a long-term goal, but you should also have small, short-term goals. These short-term goals will help you achieve the final goal quite easily.

8. Sharing is Caring

Your colleagues and friends can help you a lot in your weight loss endeavors. You should inform your colleagues about your weight loss goals and progress so that they can keep an eye on you. You can also invite them for a post-work dance class or some healthy activity. This will not only help you to lose weight but you also form a close bond with your colleagues and make your work place a happy place.

9. Get a Sipper

One of the main culprits of ruining your diet and exercise routine is craving. You have read a lot of ways to curb these cravings till now. You can also adopt a very easy way to curb the cravings in an office. You should buy a sipper and fill it with water or green tea or some other healthy and calorie-free or low-calorie drink. Whenever you feel hungry, drink from this sipper. Do not hesitate to refill it. The more you drink from this sipper, the less you will feel hungry. Staying hydrated will also keep you satiated, will curb your hunger, and will keep you active and alert as well. It will also prevent bloating, which is a side effect of consuming too much fiber without water. You can also use a simple reusable bottle if you do not have a sipper.

10. Change Your Eating Habits

It is not only eating that is important but also eating habits. There are some habits that you can adopt to enhance and help your diet routine. You should ideally sit in front of a person and eat with him or her instead of eating in front of a screen. This way, you will not eat randomly or mindlessly and instead eat properly. You should also concentrate when you are eating. You should brush your teeth after every meal so that you can avoid eating or snacking mindlessly.

11. Don't Follow Crazy Diets

A common mistake that a lot of people make when they embark on a weight loss journey is to follow a crazy diet. There seem to be a number of fad diets out there, and people fall prey to the false claims made by the promoters of these diets. However, numerous studies have shown that such fad diets can cause a lot of harm to the body and do not show long-term results, even if they help you lose weight initially.

It is actually quite easy to spot a fad diet. They promise quick results and promote some magical product or diet plan. They usually make you cut down on most of the nutritious food that your body really needs. They will probably tell you to completely cut off carbs or fats even though they are important food groups. There will be rigid rules to follow, and it will require a lot of effort on your part to follow through with such fad diets. After all, it isn't easy to drink only juice for an entire day or eat the same vegetables for the whole week. The point is, whenever you notice a diet like this, it is most likely unhealthy and ineffective.

All the weight loss tips mentioned in this book are to help you make conscious and healthy changes that will help you in the long run. It is not about following a liquid diet, fasting for days, skipping meals, or only eating soup for a month. These are the kind of crazy diets that most people try at some point or the other when they want to lose weight fast. Many times, you might see a drop in your weight after a week of following this type of diet, but it will definitely come back on sooner rather than later. Many such crazy diets will prevent you from providing your body with the nutrition that it really needs. Eating carrots or having cabbage soup for a week will not benefit your body in any way. You don't have to skip meals and stick to a single meal a day, either. In fact, this kind of diet plan sets you up for failure. You will soon be hungry and tired beyond measure. It will make you lean back on your old unhealthy habits and eat more to make up for the hunger. If you skip your timely meals, you will experience untimely cravings that will just cause more weight gain. You don't have to go on a juice cleanse to lose weight either. Homemade juices and smoothies are a great addition to your healthy diet. However, you cannot substitute all your meals with them. Your body knows how to cleanse and detoxify itself if you just eat the right kind of food. Switching to liquids for too long will have a negative effect on your digestive system as well. When you try switching back to your normal solid meals after a juice cleanses, your body will have difficulty in digesting the food.

Fad diets tend to cause the following symptoms:

- You will be dehydrated. You might be happy to drop pounds as fast as possible, but it won't be a long-term weight loss. Most of the weight loss from such diets is just water loss. You are dehydrating your body at this time, and the loss of the water weight is fooling your weighing scale. This kind of rapid dieting will only cause you to gain back the weight soon after, and you will have to follow a crazy diet again.

- You will experience nausea. The dehydration and fatigue from fad diets will make you feel nauseous. You may also get headaches. Your body is telling you that it is not getting the nutrition that it needs.

- Your digestive system will be affected, and you may suffer from constipation. It will also affect your metabolism. Cutting off calories altogether will slow down your metabolism in a major way. You need a diet that prompts your metabolic system to work faster over time. You need adequate calories, carbs, protein, and fat to maintain the upkeep of your body.

- You will lose muscle. Don't follow a diet that just makes you eat less and doesn't guide you on exercise. If you diet without exercise, you will slowly be losing muscle from your body. When you lack adequate muscle tissue, your body will be unable to burn as many calories as it should. Muscle mass is important for the body and for you to lose weight. So, you have to exercise and build muscle while you follow a healthier diet.

- You will feel weak and fatigued. You will be hungry and thirsty when you follow a fad diet. You may be willing to go through this to lose weight fast, but it is a way for your body to tell you that you are doing something wrong. It will prevent you from being productive and doing any of your other tasks as well. If you starve yourself, you will be tired and won't feel like exercising. This will mean you are affecting your weight loss plan in the long run because the body needs to be active in order to burn calories.

Given that such diets are unhealthy, they will give you the same symptoms as those that you experience when you are ill. They prevent you from consuming the adequate vitamins and minerals that your body needs. So, be more aware of what any diet asks of you, and follow only one that is actually providing your body with the nutrition it needs. A balanced diet is crucial, even if you want to lose weight.

12. Walk and Talk

A lot of our daily communications and conversations now happen over the phone; some people even talk for hours altogether on phones. Instead of sitting at one place while talking on a phone, you should pick up your mobile phone and then walk around your house or a park while talking. If you talk daily for an hour on the phone, you will automatically walk for an hour, too; thus, you can have your cake and eat it, too. Caution should be taken while trying this thing though, as you should not walk and talk while you are on the streets or in a busy area because this can prove to be fatal.

We also use text messages or instant messaging services nowadays for most of our conversations. You can try doing the walk and talk thing for this as well, but unfortunately, this can lead to headaches. Instead, you should just cut the use of instant messaging; get up, leave your place, approach the person, and talk to him or her. This is obviously only possible if you are in the same building. This will not only help you to walk, but it will also make you more productive.

You should also set reminders on your phone or watch to go out for a short walk throughout the day. You need to follow these reminders very strictly though; else, they are of no use at all.

13. Do Not Focus Too Much on the Scale

Too many people are obsessed with the number on the scale. While it can be one way to measure your progress, be sure that you are also paying attention to how you feel. Once you focus on the other benefits of a healthy diet and exercise aside from weight loss, you'll remember how satisfying it is to do these things for yourself, and you can become even more motivated.

However, this does not mean that you should not have a look at the weighing scale once a week. Monitoring your weight once a week can really help you as this is one of the best ways to check your progress, and even if your progress is not huge, it will still help you to stick to your routine.

14. Make It Fun

Losing weight shouldn't feel like a chore. You can also have fun while doing it. For example, you can invite your friends to try healthy meals the next time you hang out. You can also turn exercise into a social experience, and do it with your family and friends. You can even add some friendly competition to your workouts. Engaging in fun activities increases your chances of doing these activities again.

Exercise can be made into a very activity quite easily. If you have always wanted to dance, try to pick up a dance form that is peppy, fast, and involves a lot of body movements. Hip hop, tango, tap dance, Kathak, polka, and street dancing are some common dance forms that double as good exercises. You can also pick up belly dancing if you want to tone your muscles as well. Nowadays, dance forms like Zumba, dance aerobics, musical aerobics, etc., are becoming quite popular, too.

To make dieting an interesting ordeal, you can try making a game out of your meals. Although this might seem odd, stupid, and, in a lot of cases, downright disrespectful, if you make meals more enjoyable, you can actually keep yourself on track and follow your diet routine very closely. Having competitions is a really good method to gulp down those unappetizing veggies and soups. Playing fun or soothing music while dining can also help. As said earlier, if you socialize while eating food, you can probably eat the most unappetizing meal ever without much of a problem.

15. Use Tools and Gadgets to Help You

You are blessed to have the advantage of modern technology. There are tools, gadgets, and applications that you can use to help you achieve your goals. You can use your smartphone to download running, exercise, and even healthy cooking apps. There are also gadgets, such as heart rate monitors and step counters, that can help you measure your progress. Nowadays, you can find wonderful apps for your smartphone. These apps can turn your phone into a pedometer, compass, etc. Some apps also choose the best workout music, which is very peppy, to keep you fresh and motivated for a long time. There are some innovative apps online that can actually enhance your overall exercise or walking experience with the help of virtual reality. Try to search apps online, and use them according to your needs.

16. Learn to Celebrate Each Accomplishment

There are times when the scale won't budge, no matter what you do. Instead of letting this discourage you, you should set other goals that do not include weight loss. For example, you can set a goal of completing a half-marathon or learning a new sport or dance. Celebrating each accomplishment can inspire you to stick to your program. When you achieve goals, you can reward yourself by buying something that you really want or pampering yourself for a day. Some people even treat themselves with a little portion of their favorite non-healthy food. Celebrating each little accomplishment is very helpful because it gives you something to look forward to. You will always some excitement and anticipation that will make you work harder and with more sincerity. However, always remember that if you are going to treat yourself with your favorite food, think about the portion. Do not eat too much; keep in mind that this is a treat and not a feast.

17. Put Your Excuses Away

People can find a hundred excuses not to lose weight. It might be because they don't have the time or find it too difficult. However, these excuses are primarily psychological. Common excuses include, "I do not have good exercise equipment," "I get tired when I do exercise," or "This exercise is not meant for me." All of these are just excuses, and nothing else. There are numerous ways by which a person can successfully lose weight without fancy equipment or expensive diet pills. It is said that man is the biggest critic of himself. Make sure that you suppress your inner critic, and find a way to overcome your excuses. You should learn to motivate yourself all the time, and avoid demoralizing yourself. Do not make any excuses because excuses are double-edged swords. Not only do they prevent you from doing your exercise routine or following your diet now, but they also have psychological effect that can ruin your future weight loss plans and routine.

18. Tackling Necessary Restaurant Visits

Sometimes, you simply cannot avoid going to a restaurant and eating out. These are mostly the social occasions that are unavoidable because of their importance, such as a boss's birthday, etc. However, this does not mean that you have to break your regime and forget about your diet. You can easily avoid the foods that can ruin your diet and actually continue with your diet even in the restaurant. You can do this in the following ways:

- If you are supposed to go to a fast-food joint and cannot avoid it at all costs, you should get a vegetable burger instead of a meat burger. More often than not, veggie burgers have less calories and are healthier than the meat ones.

- If you are supposed to go to a high-quality restaurant, then you should visit its website. Nowadays, a lot of restaurants upload their menus online with complete details of each of their dishes, including the calorie count, nutrients, etc. If you plan ahead and order your researched dishes when you go to the restaurant, you can avoid eating high-calorie products. Keeping these healthy options in mind can help you to keep high calories at bay while continuing with your diet effectively.

- If you are supposed to go to a restaurant that has no website or does not upload its menu, you should ask others about it. If you are not comfortable in doing so, you should only order things that are baked, boiled, grilled, broiled, steamed, blackened, etc., and never things that are fried or breaded. Even shallow fried things should be avoided.

- You should also eat something before going out to a restaurant. Eating something healthy, such as a handful of almonds, before going out to eat will actually help you to avoid overeating.

- Eat salad, and you can do so to start your every meal every time. It will help fill you up and help you eat less of

- More often than not, the proportion of calories in a dish increases because of condiments, sauces, etc., so when you go to a restaurant, you should ideally ask for all the sauces, condiments, dressings, etc., on the side so that you can add them according to your taste. These dressings can even make a simple salad very fatty, so remember this tip always.

- If you are supposed to go to a fast-food joint or even in a restaurant, order baked potatoes with skin instead of French fries. Eat the skin as well.

- Entrée is normally served on a bed of pasta, mashed potatoes, or something similar. Instead of this, you can ask the waiter to serve it on a bed of greens, onions or something similar. This is a very healthy alternative.

- If you love wine and simply cannot resist it when you are in a restaurant, order single glasses instead of a bottle.

- Do not worry; you do not have to skip your dessert. You can always enjoy dessert, but instead of eating a complete desert, try and share it or split it. You can also order a large desert and then share it with your whole party.

Losing weight and achieving your ideal body are only half the battle. Weight maintenance can be just as difficult as losing excess weight. There are many examples of people who have lost weight very quickly but gained it back even more quickly. This happens because people go back to their original gluttonous and unhealthy lifestyle as soon as they lose weight and achieve their target. Losing weight is not a process that ends; it is a lifelong, prolonged process. You need to follow some rules throughout your life if you want to stay fit, healthy, and active. These rules are not hard to follow, and anyone with a little motivation and determination can adhere to them quite easily.

Remember, the key to maintaining your ideal weight is to keep up the lifestyle, diet, and exercise habits that you have adopted while still trying to lose weight. You obviously do not need to follow the steps that seem too difficult when you were trying to lose weight, but you should definitely follow the steps that are highly important and essential to lose weight and keep it off.

19. Patience Matters

Even while you apply these lifestyle changes, patience will matter. It can be difficult at first, but following a healthy lifestyle is much easier than you might think. You will be a little reluctant and even uncomfortable with changing your eating, exercising, and living habits at first, but this is necessary. If you are truly motivated to lose the excess weight, get fit, and take control of your body again, you must put in the effort. Focus on combining healthy eating with a more active lifestyle. Don't laze around if you want to burn more fat. Make small changes that you can follow all your life to stay healthy. Be patient, and don't rush yourself with some drastic changes. Eat all your meals, but reduce the size of your portions. Stop eating once you feel sated. You don't have to keep on eating until you feel full. Don't berate yourself for being unable to skip meals because you shouldn't be doing that in the first place. Be patient, even while you are eating your food, and savor it. Eating too quickly and not chewing will make you eat more than you need. Wait for all the scheduled meal times before you eat again. Don't expect yourself to make all the changes at once. It takes a little time to be really consistent with such things. However, if you stick to a healthy morning routine, exercise regularly, eat a balanced diet on time, and rest well, you will soon see the results of your patience and persistence. Slow down, and don't rush things; you are aiming for long-term changes for an improved body and life.

20. Understand the Reason

It is easy to read about all the healthy habits and changes that you should be making in your life. You may even motivate yourself at first to follow through with all of it. However, you won't be able to do it for long if you don't understand the reason for all of these changes. There is a reasoning behind all of the changes that you are being asked to make. There is a reason for everything that you should do. You also have to find the real reason behind why you want to embark on this weight loss journey in the first place. Think of how being overweight and unfit affects your mind, body, and life in general. Consider all the benefits of making some small lifestyle and diet changes to counteract any of the negativity associated with excess weight. Your body will be much healthier, and your mind will be sharper and happier as well. When you understand the reason for everything, you are more likely to be motivated and persistent in all that you do.

Chapter 5 – 20 Tips to Maintain Weight Loss

Now that you know all the best tips to lose weight, let's talk about how you can maintain that weight loss. The weight loss journey does not end once you reach the goal weight you had aimed for. You may have lost the excess 20 pounds, but that does not mean that you can go back to your old habits. A lot of people gain back all their old weight when they fail to understand the importance of maintenance. You may be strict and persistent throughout your diet, but it is easy to fall back on old habits. You can start eating and living the way you used to when you were overweight again. This will just diminish all the progress you have made. This is why you need to learn some tips to help you keep off the excess weight and maintain a healthy body throughout your life.

1. Write Down Why Your Goals Matter

As you start on your weight loss journey and even as you continue on it, you need to remember why your end goals matter. You may have set certain goals for yourself and thus embarked on making a change in your life in terms of food, habits, and health. However, no matter how motivated you are in the beginning, it can be easy to lose sight of your goals. This is why you should try writing it down.

Make a small note to yourself about why these goals matter to you. What is the main reason that you want to make all these changes for yourself? Think of the difference it will make in your life when you manage to achieve these goals. Write them down one by one. Is it about how you look, how you feel about your health, or even about what people think of you? No reason is too big or too small. In the end, it has to be for you and how it helps you improve your life.

Once you note down the reasons for your goals, keep the list safely with you. It will be a constant reminder of why your goals matter. You may get off track during your weight loss journey or just feel demotivated. At this point, you can read your list again and remind yourself of the importance of your goals. Some people think that losing weight is just about looking better, but it is a lot more than that. Don't give up on your goal once you have set your mind on it. Remind yourself of all the reasons why you began in the first place.

2. Create Goals for the Week

Plan out your week in advance. Set aside time on your day off, and plan out the week ahead. This is important during the weight loss plan and after. It will help you stay on track and give you a sense of accomplishment when you follow through with your plan. Making a commitment is important. Don't assume that you will somehow find time during the week to get your exercise done. More often than not, you will skip your daily exercise.

If you don't have a fixed plan, you are less likely to do the things that you don't really want to do. Everyone struggles with this, so it is understandable. However, you have to take control and prevent a relapse to your old habits. Set aside time for a daily workout, and follow the plan every day. Set goals like the amount of weight you want to lose for the week or how many miles you want to run by the end of the week. If you need to lose some extra weight, set a goal for the week.

Check your weight at the end of the week to see if you met the goal by adjusting your weekly diet and activities. You can also set goals like deciding what kind of meals you will be having the whole week. If you tend to eat out quite often, take the initiative and try to avoid a single meal outside for the whole week. Eating home-cooked food is always a healthier alternative and will facilitate weight management. When you eat out, you cannot control all the ingredients or the method of cooking for your food. So, setting such small goals for yourself will be very helpful. You have to be focused if you want to stay committed to the goals of weight loss.

Changing your habits will require consistent physical and mental energy. So, make plans to address any other stresses in your life that aggravate your unhealthy habits as well. This will improve your ability to focus on managing your habits and weight. Your goals should be realistic and focused on the week. Dealing with one small thing at a time will be possible without too much stress. As you keep completing your weekly goals, you will find it easier to continue the weight management for a longer time. Think of the process, as well as the outcome, when you set your goals.

3. Chain Your Events and Goals

Link your weight loss goals and any other events together. When you create a schedule or plan for yourself, it will allow you to do so. No matter how busy you are, there can always be time. You just have to make the time. Your event schedule might be erratic and unpredictable at times, but you can still adjust your goals to accommodate them. It is not necessary to work out at the exact same time every single day. If you know that you will have some work at the time that you usually workout, then sneak a workout in when you are free that day.

It is understandable to skip a workout when you really have no option. However, if you skip from one day to another, you are just going back to your old ways. If you don't manage your time and goals in the appropriate way, you will be unable to achieve any of the goals you have set for yourself. If your goal is to eat healthier, don't eat junk food just because it is a business lunch. You can easily order something healthy off the menu. Most restaurants will accommodate any simple adjustments to their dishes as well. If you want to consume fewer carbohydrates, make the right switches.

When you eat a hamburger, ask them to give you the patty with some greens and without the buns. Instead of mayonnaise, you can ask for a lighter dressing. Such simple requests are usually accepted by restaurants if you don't make any unreasonable demands. This way, you are sticking to healthy eating even when you eat out. If your goal is to stick to a particular calorie count, use online apps to check how many calories a certain dish has when you eat out. It is actually much easier than you would expect it to be. So, plan it all out.

If you are the one hosting such lunches out, you can do your research and find a restaurant that has really healthy food for you, too. Similarly, make an effort to chain your new lifestyle in with your other commitments. Don't use excuses to back out of what you have decided to do for yourself.

4. Follow a Consistent Routine

Building your own fitness habit can take a long time. This habit becomes easier to sustain if you have a consistent pattern. For example, you can choose to work out in the morning before going to work. Waking up at a specific time each day can condition your body to adapt to the pattern and make it easier for you to form this habit. You can always mix up the activities, but try to maintain a consistent time pattern. Make sure you stick to this even if you do not feel motivated to work out for the day. Remember, constant vigilance is the best motto for everyone who is trying to lose weight.

5. Use a Plan that Works for You

There are a lot of diets in the world, but the best is the one that you can maintain for a long period of time. Everyone has his or her own preference. Do not force yourself into a lifestyle that does not feel natural. Look for a plan that you can maintain for the long term. If you cannot honestly see yourself giving up carbohydrates, then look for a diet that provides flexibility. With this, if you plan a diet according to your need and body, you can actually increase the rate of weight loss without causing any problem or harm to your body.

6. Follow Your Plan

If you make a plan, you need to follow it. Don't just create a schedule and then leave it lying around. Use it to guide you through your days and weeks. It may seem boring or monotonous, but you will be grateful for the results it will give you. Following your plan will mean that you are efficient in achieving the goal you have set for yourself. If you drift from your plan too much, you will be less likely to see the results that you are aiming for. Don't assume that you will be able to make it work somehow without following a plan. There is a reason that a plan is being made in the first place. It can be easy to drift from one thing to another.

Following a schedule will keep you on track, even though you will have to exercise some self-discipline. The point of the plan is that you take time to figure out how you can best utilize your time and energy to achieve a particular goal. Once you create this plan, you just have to follow it. However, when you drift away from the plan, you have to constantly worry about what you should or should not be doing. This will most definitely sabotage your ultimate goals. When you are trying to maintain a healthy weight, create a healthy routine for yourself. This way, you will not compromise the effort that you put in to lose all the excess weight over time. So, follow your plan and maintain your health to lead a better quality of life.

7. Stay Active

You will need to maintain your current fitness level to maintain your current weight. Studies show that just by simply walking extra 2,000 steps or for about 20 minutes each day, people can successfully avoid excessive weight gain. You should ensure that you are physically active most days of the week.

Regular exercise must be a part of your healthy lifestyle. You do not just stop once you have achieved your weight goals. Do exercises that you find enjoyable so that you are more likely to stick to them. It is said that a 30-minute brisk walk a day can keep you healthy without much trouble. You should definitely try this option if you do not have much time. Even then, if you cannot take out time for a 30-minute walk, then you can always divide it into 5-minute instances.

You can also adopt some simple exercises to keep yourself active throughout the day. These exercises should be easy enough that you should be able to do them even when you are sitting in a chair. Exercises, such as breathing exercises, simple yoga, walking around your office, etc., are easy to do and will keep you active without interrupting your daily schedule.

8. Don't Skip Days

You need to understand the importance of consistency. It would have been a hard change for you when you first started working out regularly in the first place. Maybe your weight goal motivated you at the time. This might have kept you going to the gym or just working out consistently. However, many people start skipping days when they have achieved their goal. You might not have to do a hardcore workout to lose weight like you previously did, but you still need regular exercise.

If you skip days and start getting lazy, your body will stop burning calories as well. You need to maintain the new habit that you have created. You get your rest days, and maybe you can add another rest day once you have achieved your goal. But you still need to keep exercising on the other days. The intensity of the workout can be adjusted according to your goal of losing more weight or just maintaining your present weight. Professional athletes, bodybuilders, etc. do not stop working out once they have finished a race or achieved that ripped body. They continue to stay active and persist in their effort because they know that they can easily lose what they have gained.

In the same way, you can easily gain back all the weight you lost if you start slacking. The worst part is, the time it would take to gain back the weight is much shorter than the time it took you to lose it. You can have rest days every week. However, fix days for working out, and follow through with them. One skipped day can easily become two and more. Pretty soon, you will find yourself going through the same old struggle to try and get back on track. It would just be simpler to follow through with your dedicated time for a workout every week. This will allow you to enjoy the benefits of the healthy body that you have attained for yourself. Skipping your workouts will make you feel unfit from fit, faster than you can imagine. So, stick to your days if you want to keep feeling good about your body.

9. Keep Stress at Bay

Stress can push you to make unhealthy choices. Even if you eat healthy and exercise, too much stress can make you gain weight. Stress can trigger adrenalin and cortisol, which cause your body to feel hungry even if you are not. When stressed, most people have cravings for sweets, as well as high-fat and salty foods, because these foods stimulate the brain to produce pleasure-inducing chemicals that can counteract the tension experienced by the body.

Moving your body is an effective stress reliever. It can aid your blood circulation while enabling cortisol to be flushed out of your body. You should also do activities that you find relaxing on a regular basis to prevent stress from accumulating.

Stress can also enhance the problems that are considered to be the side effects of obesity. Stress can lead to problems of the heart, brain, and nervous system. Sometimes, people are stressed about their extra weight, but as said above, stress can actually lead to weight gain; thus, this forms a vicious cycle. To break free of this cycle, you need to cope with stress effectively. Meditation and yoga are highly effective in controlling and countering stress. You should try breathing exercises and

Pranayama as well. These few things will help you a lot to control stress.

10. Sleep Well

The body needs a proper amount of rest to function well. Proper amounts of sleep can also help replenish your energy and help your muscles recover from your workouts. Make sure that your bedroom is conducive for sleeping. Condition yourself to see your bedroom as a place for sleeping and relaxation. Moreover, it is better if you do not rely on stimulants to control your sleeping patterns because these chemicals can become addictive and may cause you to become dependent on them. It is highly advised to get at least six to seven hours of sleep every night. This sleep will keep you active, rested, and healthy.

11. Avoid Unplanned Eating and Drinking

Eating unplanned meals can cause you to overeat. Make sure that you schedule snacks throughout the day to manage your hunger. Planning your meals can also ensure that you are eating a well-balanced diet. This enables you to have all of the nutrients that you need to keep your body energized and healthy. You should also mix up your meals every week so that you don't get bored eating the same foods each day. A boring and repetitive diet can prove to be a great challenge and problem if you are trying to lose weight, so keep it fun.

12. Plan and Set Reminders

A planner or online calendar can keep you organized. You can schedule your workouts and treat them just like any other business appointment. You can also place reminders and motivations in a place where you can easily see them. Reading a few words of encouragement can spark your motivation. You can even create your own motivational board. Cut out pictures, quotes, or anything that can inspire you. Stick them on a wall or cork board. Nowadays, everyone has a smartphone, and there are many apps available online that can help you to track your routine and set reminders as well. Use these apps effectively, as they are free of any hassles and are extremely user-friendly and easy to use.

13.   Make Sure You Have a Healthy Perspective on Food

Food is the main fuel for our bodies. Emotional eating can be described as using food to escape from your problems. Certain foods may trigger the release of feel-good hormones in the body but do not actually make everything okay. Be aware of the real reasons why you overeat or crave unhealthy foods. Avoid eating for the wrong reasons. Keep a log of the instances in which you ate for reasons other than hunger. You should also maintain the good eating habits that you have established when you were still losing weight. It is extremely important to understand that losing weight alone is not important; what is more important is maintaining the lost weight. Some people lose weight easily but struggle to maintain the lost weight. If you are one of these people, try hard to keep weight at bay.

14.   Maintain a Positive Mindset

Negativity can only make you feel bad. Remember that a healthy lifestyle is about balance. Do not be depressed if you fail once in a while. This does not mean that all of your efforts are wasted. Just do your best to get back on track. Finding your own methods of maintaining weight can make you feel good about your accomplishments. Dwelling on positive thoughts can also motivate you. As said above, losing weight is not at all about physical strength and power; it is more about how mentally strong you are. If you keep your mind healthy and active, you will lose weight in no time.

15. Fuel Your Body Before and After Workouts

It is advisable to have a snack or workout shake before and after exercising. Choose a snack or shake that is rich in good carbohydrates and protein. Such foods can increase the flow of amino acid into your muscles and stimulate muscle growth and strength. It is particularly important that you nourish your body after workouts to prevent starvation and fatigue. Do not choose any fatty or unhealthy snack. These snacks are not only unhealthy for you, but they provide low to zero nutrition. Ask your dietician or check online for snacks that are healthy, full of nutrition, and can be consumed without any problems as such.

16. Be Inspired; Don't Compare

You are not the only person struggling with weight issues. A large percentage of people around the world have faced weight-related issues at some point in their life. The modern-day diet and lifestyle are some of the main causes of obesity in people of our generation. If you look up weight loss stories, you will find many inspirational people who have worked hard to turn their life around. You need to find inspiration from them, and keep going.

You may even notice your workout buddy or other people in the gym making progress. This can be quite intimidating for most people, especially when your personal progress is quite slow. However, remember that everybody is different. If someone else is losing weight and getting more fit, you should focus on finding inspiration from them. Don't envy them and demotivate yourself. Try to learn if they are doing something different that might help you as well. You can use them as your guide to improve yourself. A lot of these people will be very willing to help you out, too.

Don't compare your body and progress to someone else's. They are a completely different person, and weighing less does not make them better than you. When you start on a weight loss journey with someone else, it may seem natural to compare your progress with the other person's. This is especially true when you are both doing the exact same thing, but the other person is making better progress. However, you have to understand that there can be different reasons for this. His or her metabolism might just naturally be faster than yours. Do not let this be a reason for you to berate yourself and give up.

Comparison can actually do more harm than good. You don't need to try and become the same dress size as the other person. People lose and gain weight at different rates, and bodies will always be uniquely different from each other. Don't focus on how unfair it is that another person is losing more weight when you are working just as hard, if not more. Use their progress as inspiration, and just keep working toward your own goals. Inspiration will be a more positive influence than comparison. Accept yourself throughout the process.

17. Words Can Be Inspiring

Have you noticed how motivated you feel when someone reassures you or gives you a good talk? Words have a power of their own. This is why you should consider the power of words in keeping you inspired to lose extra pounds and maintain a healthy weight. We all have a voice in our head that sometimes tells us just to give up, especially when we are doing something that we don't necessarily like or enjoy. Exercising and eating healthy food is not usually as easy as some people make it out to be. It is much easier to eat sugary foods and laze around watching movies. However, you have to ignore the voice telling you to give up and instead listen to the quieter voice that is telling you to keep going.

Whenever you feel a lack of motivation, you should find a way to be inspired. You can ask someone to talk to you and motivate you again. This can be your workout buddy, instructor, family, or just a friend who has seen you work toward your weight loss goals. They will remind you of all your hard work and why you started in the first place. Otherwise, you can just look up some inspirational quotes and keep yourself motivated. Print out some inspirational quotes, and stick them on your desk, locker, wardrobe, gym, or anywhere that will force you to read them. They will be a regular reminder to keep going on your journey.

You can also download a lot of motivational quotes and save them as the wallpaper on your phone or laptop. Seeing these words often will give you more strength. This will prevent you from relapsing into your old habits and destroying the progress you have made. It is actually quite easy to find motivational quotes specifically meant for weight loss. You can also listen to podcasts by people who have gone through the same things as you. Listening to people talk about their journey and how they made progress can help you keep going. Words can be very inspiring when you are feeling completely defeated and on the verge of giving up.

18. Imagine Your Success

Visualize. Imagine yourself achieving the weight loss goals that you have set for yourself. Think of the weighing scale showing the number you want it to. Imagine how you will look in the dress you want to wear to the next party. Visualization can be a powerful tool in your journey. It will show you what you have to look forward to. It will give you a reason to keep going. Imagine succeeding in achieving your goals. Think of the gratification you will experience once you reach that point. The power of visualization is more underrated than it should be. Even before you begin your weight loss plan, you should try visualization.

Get into your mind, and shift the negative mental image that you have of yourself. Don't think of yourself as an overweight and unattractive person because you aren't. However, to motivate yourself to achieve a particular weight loss goal, you can try imagining yourself at that weight. Think of how you will look when you lose the extra pounds and how much happier you will be at that point. Imagine yourself as a fit and successful person. Use this mental image to fuel your persistence in losing weight. This mental trick can be very effective in helping you accept all the hard work that you will have to do along the way. It will make you feel as though all the hard work is worth it, and you will be less willing to give up midway.

Your mind doesn't really know the difference between what you are imagining and what is real. This is why your subconscious will somehow imagine that mental image of yourself as something that has already happened. This kind of visualization has helped many successful people in different fields to build more confidence and attain more success. Studies have shown that this kind of visualization technique has helped many people develop healthy habits and get fit. People who use this trick may even see better results in a shorter time as compared to those who don't try it. You can try this when you wake up in the morning or just before you fall asleep at night. Relax and calm your mind as you picture yourself as you want to be.

Imagine yourself doing all the exercises you should be doing and eating only healthy food. Notice how you feel during all this and try to connect with your emotions. Let this exercise internalize these images. Doing this regularly can be extremely helpful, and you will see how much easier it is for you to follow through with your weight loss plan.

19. Compete with the Past You

If you are aiming for a change in your life, there is always a reason for it. If you are trying to lose weight, you probably have a reason for wanting the change. Most people with weight issues have trouble accepting themselves and face numerous issues associated with excess weight. So, when you are trying to build a new you, compete with the older version of yourself that you were not happy with. Don't repeat the same mistakes that you did before. By now, you should be aware of what you did wrong and how you can do much better.

Motivate yourself to do better than you did before. You are working towards improving yourself, so you cannot afford to be less than what you were before. If you were lazy and avoided physical exercise before, you have to push yourself to be more active. Even if you used to go for a walk, increase your timing compared to before. If you had bad eating habits, work on improving them little by little. Avoid eating sweets or junk food that you used to eat too much off. Don't sit for too long, and avoid binge eating when you are bored or feeling too emotional.

Just try to do better in everything you did before. Think of how much better you will feel about yourself when you see real progress. Everyone can be a better version of themselves at any point in their lives. However, this will require effort and persistence. Don't fall back on old habits that will make you go through the same unhealthy experience again. In your weight loss journey, you can continuously make an effort to do better than the previous day.

While running, try to increase your pace or your timing a little more than the last time. Add an extra workout day as compared to the previous week. Control your portions a little better than you did before. You will surely see significant progress in your weight loss journey in this way.

There are many ways in which you can challenge yourself or compete with yourself:

- Place a bet. Bet on yourself about something like how much weight you can lose in a certain period of time. You can bet using an app with a friend or just by yourself. It could be money, or it could be a treat you allow yourself if you win the bet. It doesn't have to be some drastic change or an unhealthy ultimatum. Set a reasonable bet on how much you could easily lose in a couple of weeks. When you win the bet, you will be motivating yourself to keep going and rewarding yourself.

- Make a pact. Make a pact with yourself about doing something different. It could be about going to the gym more regularly than before. Make a pact that you will go to the gym five days a week, no matter what, for two months. Strive to keep this pact with yourself. It could also be about including fresh vegetables in all your meals to eat healthier. Keep a log of these activities to make sure that you stick to your pact.

20. Be Patient

If you are aiming for permanent weight loss, you have to work toward reaching the ideal weight and then maintaining it. Patience is a very important factor in case you want long-term weight loss. If you are not patient, you will probably be making decisions that give you short-term results and leave you disappointed in the long run. Shortsighted decisions are usually associated with diets that are too restrictive; this typically happens when you want to see instant results. This kind of approach will leave you feeling deprived, and at some point, you will resume all your old eating habits.

You might restrict your calories to an unhealthy level, and this can leave you fatigued, nauseous, and feeling ill. This is why you need a dieting approach that will be moderate and give you long-term results. You have to think and plan as you create a weight loss plan that is sustainable for you. Think of the various elements that will give you a sound weight loss plan that ensures success in the long run.

If you stick to your weight loss plan, you will probably be successful in achieving your goals. You have to be patient throughout the process and even after it. Don't assume that your work is done once you lose the extra pounds. Working to maintain this ideal weight can also be quite challenging for most people. You might have expected that the hard part would only have been to lose the weight. You still can't eat as you please and stop exercising altogether. However, you can definitely go a little easier on yourself. Your workouts can be a little less strenuous, and you can allow yourself some unhealthy treats once in a while.

You may even see your weight increase a little sometimes. Don't get anxious or impatient about this. You can easily regain control again. Just be more conscious about what you put on your plate, and don't let your portions be larger than what your body actually needs. People tend to lose patience quite fast, and this applies during the cycle of weight loss. The time it takes to lose the extra pounds off your body will be like a learning period for you. You will understand what your body needs and how it reacts to different things. What you learn in this period will be useful for when you struggle to maintain the new body you have gained. It is not just about what you eat and how much you exercise.

Your attitude toward it all and how you face different challenges play a very important role. Take your time to understand your body, and be patient through it all. Practicing patience will allow you to be successful and motivate you to get back up even when you face a problem. Identify the healthy habits that make you feel good about yourself, and keep repeating them. When something doesn't work out, learn from it, and do something new. Don't let any criticism from other people affect you. Build your confidence, and be patient with yourself. Celebrate your victories, and learn from your failures along the way.

Chapter 6 – 12 Bonus Recipes to Get on with Your Diet

Up to this point, we have seen a lot of tips that can help you to lose weight very effectively. In this chapter, we have included some really easy-to-make and very tasty recipes that will help you with your diet and exercise routines.

Pizza Crust Made of Quinoa

Calories – 90

Carbs – 13 g

Protein – 2 g

Fat – 5 g

Ingredients

- Quinoa, washed and drained, ¾ cup
- Water, ¼ cup
- Salt, ½ teaspoon
- Baking Powder, 1 teaspoon
- Oil, 1 tablespoon (coconut or olive oil recommended)

Method

1. Wash and rinse the quinoa. Let it dry.
2. In a bowl, put in the quinoa, and soak it in some water. Keep it in water for at least 8 hours.

3. When quinoa has been soaked, set the oven on 425 degrees.
4. Rinse the quinoa once again, and then let it dry thoroughly on a towel.
5. In a food processor add the salt, the water, baking powder and finally the quinoa. Process it until you get a thick paste.
6. In a deep baking dish, spread the layer of this paste. You need to oil the pan first.
7. Bake the pizza for 15 minutes, and then turn it over after taking it out.
8. Once again, bake it for around 5 minutes.
9. Take the pizza out, and add your favorite ingredients on top. Bake for around 5 minutes more.
10. Serve hot or cold.

Creamy Thai Soup

Calories – 137

Carbs – 14 g

Protein – 5 g

Fat – 6 g

Ingredients

- Green onions, chopped
- Gluten-free vegetable/chicken stock, 2 cups
- Sun butter, 1 cup
- Garlic, minced, 1 clove
- Ginger, grated or minced, 1-inch piece
- Gluten-free soy sauce, 1 tablespoon
- Honey, 1 teaspoon
- Juice of 1 lime
- Coconut milk, 1 cup
- Red pepper flakes

Method

1. Chop the white part of the green onions. Blend it.
2. Add all the other ingredients and blend until smooth.
3. Cook this blended mixture in a medium-sized pan on medium heat.
4. Serve hot with red pepper flakes.

Green Pea and Parsley Soup

Calories – 210

Carbs – 36 g

Protein – 13 g

Fat – 3 g

Ingredients

- Coconut oil
- Onions, 2 (medium sized)
- Garlic, 4 cloves
- Sea Salt
- Parsley leaves, 2 cups
- Vegetable broth, 3–4 cups
- Lemon juice, 1 tablespoon
- Olive oil, 1 tablespoon
- Peas, ½ kg
- Zest of ½ lemon

Method

1. Chop garlic and onions.
2. In a large pot, heat oil and sauté garlic, onion, salt.
3. Pour in the broth and then the peas. Let it cook. After this, add the parsley. Cook once again. Blend this in a mixer until smooth.
4. Add zest, lemon juice, and oil. Blend this once again.
5. Season with salt, etc., and garnish with parsley.

Stuffed Sweet Potatoes

Calories – 307

Carbs – 53 g

Protein – 15 g

Fat – 5 g

Ingredients

- Sweet potatoes, small, 4
- Olive oil, 1 teaspoon
- Red onion, small, 1
- Garlic, 1 clove
- Cumin powder, 1 teaspoon
- Chilli powder, ½ teaspoon
- Tomatoes, 1 can, chopped
- Black beans, cooked, ½ cup
- Frozen corn kernels, ½ cup
- Chopped cilantro
- Sea salt and ground pepper, to taste

Method

1. Keep oven on preheat mode at 400 F. Bake the sweet potatoes until they are done. Poke them with a fork to get them done faster. You can also microwave them.
2. While the sweet potatoes are getting done, in a medium skillet, soften some onions with olive oil. Next, add garlic, and cook more.
3. To the above mixture, add chili, cumin, and salt and then mix.

4. Add tomatoes, beans, and corn and sauté. Finally, add cilantro, salt, and pepper.
5. When the sweet potatoes are done, take them out of the oven, and slice them down the middle. Season them with salt and pepper, and pour the filling over them.
6. Serve hot.

Baked Paleo Chicken

Calories – 200

Carbs – 0 g

Protein – 41.5 g

Fat – 4.8 g

Ingredients

- Chicken tenderloins, 2 pounds
- Blanched almond flour, 1 cup
- Flax meal, 1 tablespoon
- Paprika, 1 teaspoon
- Garlic powder, ½ teaspoon
- Sea salt, ½ teaspoon
- Dried parsley, ½ teaspoon
- Poultry seasoning, ¼ teaspoon
- Black pepper, ground
- Eggs, 2
- Olive oil spray

Method

1. Keep oven on preheat mode at 425 F, and line two large baking trays with baking paper.
2. In a bowl, add flour, garlic powder, flax meal, paprika sea salt, poultry seasoning, parsley, and pepper.
3. Beat the eggs in a bowl.
4. Coat the chicken with the eggs. Dredge them in the flour mix.

5. Oil the baking sheets, and place the chicken tenders. Bake for 10 minutes, flip spray the oil and bake for another 10 minutes at around 180 F.
6. Serve hot.

Brunch Banana Pancakes

Calories – 78

Carbs – 10 g

Protein – 1.8 g

Fat – 3.5 g

Ingredients

1. Bananas, large and overripe, 2
2. Baking powder, 1/8 teaspoon
3. Eggs, 2
4. Topping of your choice

Method

1. Take a large bowl, and beat eggs with baking powder.
2. Take another bowl, and mash bananas in it.
3. Mix the ingredients of both the bowls in another bowl.
4. Take a frying pan, and make small pancakes. Make at least 10 pancakes with the batter.
5. Serve hot.

Hawaiian Chicken Salad

Calories – 227.3

Carbs – 22 g

Protein – 11 g

Fat – 10.9 g

Ingredients

For the salad

- Shredded cooked chicken, 3 cups
- Chopped green cabbage, 1 cup
- Chopped cilantro/parsley, ¼ cup
- Green onions, finely chopped, ¾ cup
- Fresh chopped pineapple, ½ cup
- Silvered almond, toasted lightly ¼ cup

For the dressing

- Chopped fresh pineapple, ¼ cup
- Lime juice, 1 tablespoon
- Honey, 1 tablespoon
- Fresh ginger root, 1 piece
- Extra virgin olive oil, 1 tablespoon
- Salt
- Black pepper
- Coconut aminos, 2 tablespoons
- Lime zest

Method

1. Blend all the ingredients of the dressing portion in a blender, and blend until it becomes a smooth paste.
2. In a bowl, add all the salad ingredients and toss.
3. Add the dressing to this bowl, and toss once again.
4. Season with salt, pepper, and lime zest.

Vegan Risotto

Calories – 433.5

Carbs – 7.7 g

Protein – 1 g

Fat – 6.9 g

Ingredients

- Olive oil, 1 tablespoon
- Dairy-free margarine, 1 tablespoon
- Garlic, minced, 2 cloves
- White onion, chopped, ¼ cup
- Arborio rice, 2 cups
- Salt
- Ground pepper
- Veggie broth, warm, 6 cups
- White wine, warm, 1 cup
- Zucchini, grated, small, 2
- Diced mushrooms, ½ cup
- Chopped broccoli, 1 cup
- Yeast, 1 tablespoon
- Sun-dried tomatoes, chopped, 2 cups
- Dairy-free margarine, 2 tablespoons
- Basil, chopped, 2 tablespoons

Method

1. In a large pan, heat margarine and oil. Sauté some garlic and onion in it. Add the rice to this pan, and then add the salt and pepper. Let it cook for a bit. Finally add the broth. Let it boil.

2. When the liquid starts reducing, add the wine slowly. Add the vegetables when almost all the wine is used.
3. Remove from heat. Put in margarine, yeast, basil, and tomatoes.
4. Serve hot.

Moo Shu Beef

Calories – 492

Carbs – 48 g

Protein – 34 g

Fat – 18 g

Ingredients

- Top sirloin steak, 1 pound
- Shiitake mushrooms, thinly sliced, ½ cup
- Bean sprouts, ½ cup
- Green cabbage, thinly sliced, 1/2 head
- Carrot, thinly sliced, 1

For the Marinade

- Gluten-free soy sauce, 2 tablespoons
- Dark sesame oil, 1 tablespoon
- Water, 2 tablespoons
- Granulated sugar, 1 tablespoon
- Garlic cloves, minced, 3

For the Sauce

- Gluten-free soy sauce, 2 tablespoons
- Dark sesame oil, 1 tablespoon
- Ground ginger, 1/4 teaspoon
- Granulated sugar, 2 teaspoons
- Water, 2 teaspoons
- Green onion, sliced thinly, 1

- Onion powder, 1/4 teaspoon
- Ground black pepper, 1/2 teaspoon
- Garlic powder, 1/4 teaspoon
- Water, 3 tablespoons
- Cornstarch, 2 teaspoons

Method

1. Take a bowl, and add all ingredients for the marinade. In another bowl, mix all the ingredients for the sauce, except for the cornstarch and water. In another bowl, make slurry of cornstarch and water.
2. Cut the steaks, and marinate them.
3. Heat oil in a skillet, and then cook some steak in it. Now, add the veggies. Let it cook for a bit, and finally, add the slurry.
4. Cook until done.
5. Serve hot over rice.

Nicholas Bjorn

Amaranth salad

Calories – 251

Carbs – 46 g

Protein – 9.4 g

Fat – 3.9 g

Ingredients

- Cold water, 1 ½ cups
- Uncooked whole-grain amaranth, ½ cup
- Chopped fresh mint, ¼ cup
- Extra-virgin olive oil, 2 tablespoons
- Grated lemon rind, 1 teaspoon
- Pine nuts, toasted, ¼ cup
- Diced unpeeled English cucumber, 2 cups
- Thinly sliced celery, ½ cup
- Chopped fresh flat-leaf parsley, ¼ cup
- Finely chopped red onion, ½ cup
- Fresh lemon juice, 2 tablespoons
- Salt
- Crushed red pepper, ¼ teaspoon
- Canned chickpeas, drained, ½ cup
- Feta cheese, crumbled, 1 cup
- Lemon wedges

Method

1. Boil amaranth in cold water in a sauce pan. Do this on medium heat. Cook until the amaranth absorbs all of the water.

2. Take a bowl, and add everything in it except the cheese and the lemon. Toss.
3. Rinse amaranth under cold running water. Do this in a sieve.
4. In the bowl, add the amaranth and then mix everything together. Serve with lemon wedges and cheese.

Risotto Soup

Calories – 320

Carbs – 46.2 g

Protein – 14.9 g

Fat – 7.5 g

Ingredients

- Olive oil, 1 tablespoon
- Chopped onion, 2 cups
- Grated lemon rind, 2 teaspoons
- Arborio rice, 3/4 cup
- Spinach, coarsely chopped, 2 cups
- Ground nutmeg, ¼ tsp
- Parmesan cheese, grated, ½ cup
- Less-sodium chicken broth, 2 cans
- Asparagus, sliced, 2 cups

Method

1. Take a large sauce pan, and sauté some onions in olive oil. Do this on medium heat. Next, put in the rind and the rice. Sauté once again.
2. Gradually add the broth, and let it simmer. Keep a lid on the pan. Simmer for around 10 minutes.
3. Put in the asparagus and the spinach. Add nutmeg, and cook the broth uncovered.
4. Serve hot when done, and top it with cheese.

Tuna Salad

Calories – 190.3

Carbs – 11.7 g

Protein – 32.3 g

Fat – 2.2 g

Ingredients

- Albacore tuna, 1 can
- Non-fat cottage cheese, 3/4th cup
- Low fat yogurt, 4 tbsp
- Chopped red onion, ¼ cup
- Celery stalk, 1
- Dijon mustard, 1 teaspoon
- Lemon juice
- Dill

Method

1. Take a large salad bowl, and add the tuna in.
2. Then, add the yogurt and cottage cheese, and mix with the tuna.
3. Add the chopped onion and celery.
4. Add a splash of lemon juice, Dijon mustard, and some dill to finish preparing the salad.

Nicholas Bjorn

Conclusion

Thank you again for choosing this book! I sincerely hope that you received value from it.

I really hope that this book was able to help teach you how to lose weight effectively and permanently. Consistency and constant vigilance are necessary to lose weight and to keep it at bay. It is all about mental strength and power. Losing weight is not important, but losing weight in a healthy way is. You should also try and strive hard to maintain your body.

The next step is to follow the methods listed in this book, and apply what you have just learned. Take action, and be consistent!

Finally, if you enjoyed this book, then I'd like to ask you for a favor, would you be kind enough to leave a review for this audio book? It'd be greatly appreciated! I want to reach as many people as I can with this book and more reviews will help me accomplish that!

Thank you and good luck!

FREE E-BOOKS SENT WEEKLY

Join North Star Readers Book Club
And Get Exclusive Access To The Latest Kindle Books in Health, Fitness, Weight Loss and Much More…

TO GET YOU STARTED HERE IS YOUR FREE E-BOOK:

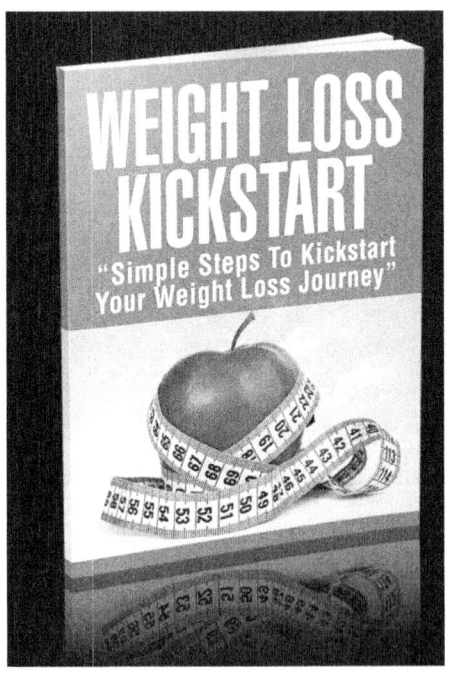

Visit to Sign Up Today!
www.northstarreaders.com/weight-loss-kick-start

GOOD NUTRITION IS IMPORTANT – THIS IS A FACT.

BUT HOW DO YOU REALLY GET STARTED TO ACHIEVING IT? PEOPLE SAY IT BEGINS WITH A BALANCED DIET, BUT HOW EXACTLY DO YOU ACHIEVE THAT BALANCE?

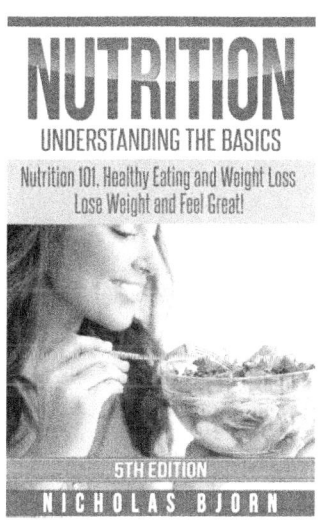

If you are lost in the world of calories and kilojoules, this book is the perfect reference to help you! The contents of this book will help you focus on what's important while getting rid of all the unnecessary fluff about dieting and healthy living that are just bound to confuse you.

Here is what this book has in store for you:
- Nutrition defined and simplified
- Dietary guidelines made easy to follow
- Nutrition labels made understandable
- Vitamins and minerals explained
- Fat-burning foods enumerated
- Meal planning and recipes made doable

Start reaping the benefits of eating healthy and living healthy! You can get started today.

Visit to Order Your Copy Today!
https://www.amazon.com/dp/1519485492

DO YOU WANT TO KNOW HOW YOU CAN LOSE WEIGHT AND BUILD MUSCLE FAST, STARTING RIGHT NOW? THIS BOOK WILL LET YOU IN ON THE SECRET!

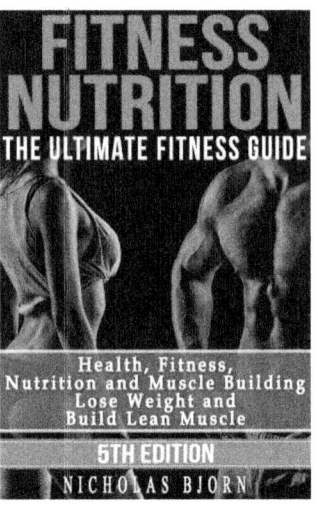

Everyone knows how important it is to maintain a healthy physique. Often, achieving the ideal body requires you to lose weight and build lean muscle. But how do you do that? To become physically fit, you need to have the knowledge necessary to get you on your way and the motivation required to keep you going.

Here's what this book has in store for you:
- Learn how your body uses calories and what role carbohydrates play in your weight
- Discover which foods contain good fats and lean protein that could benefit your body
- Determine what your meal frequency and caloric intake should be
- Know which exercises you should do to get that toned and sculpted look

With the knowledge you will gain from this book, you will be on your way to getting the amazing body that you want!

Visit to Order Your Copy Today!
https://www.amazon.com/dp/1514832968

Stop Dieting

How to Stop Dieting and Eat Normally

The Best Healthy Weight Loss Foods to Eat

3rd Edition

By Nicholas Bjorn

Nicholas Bjorn

© Copyright 2020 – All rights reserved.

The contents of this book may not be reproduced, duplicated, or transmitted without direct written permission from the author.

Under no circumstances will any legal responsibility or blame be held against the publisher for any reparation, damages, or monetary loss due to the information herein, either directly or indirectly.

Legal Notice:

This book is copyright protected. This is only for personal use. You cannot amend, distribute, sell, use, quote, or paraphrase any part of the content within this book without the consent of the author.

Disclaimer Notice:

Please note the information contained within this document is for educational and entertainment purposes only. Every attempt has been made to provide accurate, up-to-date, complete, and reliable information. No warranties of any kind are expressed or implied. Readers acknowledge that the author is not engaging in the rendering of legal, financial, medical, or professional advice. The content of this book has been derived from various sources. Please consult a licensed professional before attempting any techniques outlined in this book.

By reading this document, the reader agrees that under no circumstances is the author responsible for any losses, direct or indirect, which are incurred as a result of the use of information contained within this document, including, but not limited to, errors, omissions, or inaccuracies.

Table of Contents

Introduction 147

Chapter 1 – 10 Nutrition Rules for Boosting Energy Burning Fat... 149

Chapter 2 – Top 10 Herbs and Spices to Help Improve Health and Weight Loss 155

Chapter 3 – 36 Fat Burning Super Foods 159

Chapter 4 - The Top 20 Superfoods You Should be Eating 171

Chapter 5 – 8 Reasons Why You Are Not Losing Body Fat 205

Chapter 6 – Eat Right For Weight Loss 211

   Basal Metabolic Rate (BMR) 212

   Metabolism and Weight Loss 214

   What Else Can I Do? 219

Chapter 7 – Planning Your Meals 225

Chapter 8 – The Importance of Water 229

   Benefits of Drinking Water..229

   How Much Water Should I Drink?.......................................234

   Water and its Many Forms 234

   The Role of Water in Weight Loss...235

Chapter 9 – Strength Training: A Vital Component of Your Weight Loss Journey..239

Chapter 10 – Kitchen Implements and Gadgets for Healthy Cooking 241

Chapter 11 – Refrigerator Essentials for Healthy Eating 245

    For Your Freezer 247

Chapter 12 – How to Eat Healthy Without Going Broke and Losing Your Mind 249

    Shopping the Right Way for Health...................................... 249

Chapter 13 – 15 Tasty Super Food Smoothies Recipes 253

    Peanut Butter Power Shake 253

    Dark Chocolate Shake 253

    CHIA Green Smoothie 254

    The Winter Mint Chocolate Shake.. 254

    Green Spinach-Apple-Mango Yogurt Smoothie 254

    Anti-Aging Kiwi-Blueberry Smoothie....................................255

    Berry Banana Smoothie 255

    Peach-Mango Yogurt Smoothie 256

    The Lean Muscle Mochaccino... 256

    Orange Creamsicle Smoothie... 256

    Liquid Breakfast Smoothie...257

Banana Nut Shake 257

Strawberry Shortcake Smoothie.. 257

Mango Pineapple Shake 258

Creamy Chocolate Avocado Smoothie..................................258

Chapter 14 – 5 Tasty Super Food Soup Recipes........ 259

Green Superfood Soup..259

Carrot and Turmeric Soup.. 261

Dairy-Free Creamy Avocado Soup 263

Spicy Chicken and Quinoa Soup...264

Slow Cooker Superfood Soup 266

Chapter 15 – 6 Yummy and Healthy One-Bowl Meals 269

Quinoa and Chicken Burrito Bowl with Green Sauce 269

French Lentil Salad with Goat Cheese 273

Thai Chicken Soup with Rice Noodles 275

Cauliflower Fried Rice 277

Thai Shrimp and Quinoa 279

Ratatouille Rice... 281

Chapter 16 – Sweet Endings: Lip Smacking Healthy Desserts 283

Avocado Chocolate Mousse with Summer Fruit 283

Raspberry Vegan Cheesecake 285

Cinnamon Baked Pears 287

Healthy Peanut Butter Fudge 288

No-Bake Brownie Energy Bites 290

Apple Crumble 291

Yogurt Cocktail 293

Quick Coffee Dessert 295

Simple Rice Pudding 297

Rich Chocolate Slices 298

Conclusion 301
References 303

Introduction

This book includes proven steps and strategies on how you can boost energy and burn fat, plus the best fat burning super foods you should be eating for healthy weight loss.

If you have tried to lose weight before, you know it's not always easy. With so many diets to choose from and each telling you're a different way to eat and what foods to avoid; it can easily get confusing or frustrating. That's why this book focuses on normal foods you can actually eat to not only lose weight, but also improve your health.

If you are truly serious about losing weight and are prepared to make the commitment to eating healthier, then this is the book for you.

FREE E-BOOKS SENT WEEKLY

Join North Star Readers Book Club
And Get Exclusive Access To The Latest Kindle Books in Health, Fitness, Weight Loss and Much More...

TO GET YOU STARTED HERE IS YOUR FREE E-BOOK:

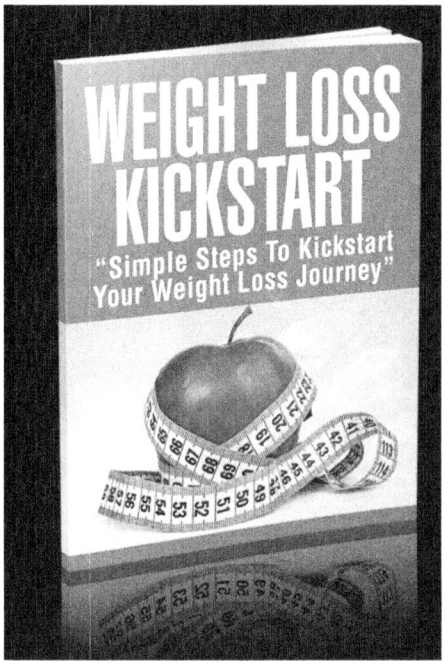

Visit to Sign Up Today!
www.northstarreaders.com/weight-loss-kick-start

Chapter 1 – 10 Nutrition Rules for Boosting Energy Burning Fat

Everyone wants to feel good, to feel alert, rested and full of energy but, for most, this is just a dream. The reality is we live in a harsh world, where time is in short supply and stress is in abundance. Lack of sleep combined with poor diet and stress leads to illness and exhaustion.

Fatigue is one of the worst things for the human body; it breaks us down emotionally and physically and it wreaks total havoc on our immune systems, which opens the way for chronic disease. But we all have the power needed to make that change, to give our bodies the energy boost they need and to feel fantastic with it.

Regular exercise, learning how to manage stress and sleeping properly are all critical factors in being able to combat fatigue but you can also make a change to your eating habits. The following are ten ways in which you can use the food you eat to give you energy that lasts throughout the day.

Rule Number 1 – Eat Foods that are Dense in Nutrients

The best way to boost your metabolism to convert your food into energy is eat foods that contain the right minerals and vitamins – and plenty of them. If you eat the right food, all the cells in your body will produce energy to keep you going.

Rule Number 2 – Eat Foods that are High in Antioxidants

These are the scavengers that clean out all the chemicals and toxins in the body that are wearing you down. Eat plenty of fruits and vegetables and other plant-based foods rather than taking them in supplement form. Eating too much of some nutrients can be risky so get round this by eating only whole foods, like colorful berries, melons and dark green leafy vegetables.

Rule Number 3 – Eating your Omega-3's

Over the years, research has shown that plenty of omega-3 in your diet can improve your memory, mood and thinking, all of which are closely related to energy. Try to eat one good helping per day in the form of flax oil or seeds, fish, hemp oil or seeds, leafy greens and walnuts.

Rule Number 4 – Stop Dieting

Most diets are no good for the human body because they require you to deprive your body of certain foods. You should not cut your calories down too much because this just decreases your metabolism. That is why many people who are on strict diets often complain of lethargy. And, as your metabolism slows down, your body will burn off less calories, which means the ultimate result, is a gain in weight. Eat the right amount of calorie needs every day and eat them in the right foods, combined with regular exercise if you want to successfully drop the pounds.

Rule Number 5 – Don't Skip Breakfast

Yes, it is so easy, when you are running late and there are those who think that to lose weight they have to skip a meal. It is the wrong meal to skip. Breakfast is the most important meal of the day as it gets your metabolism off and running and a good breakfast will keep your energy levels up until it's time for lunch. Instead of hitting the bagel bar or eating stodgy cereals, go for eggs, fresh fruit, whole grain cereal and nuts.

Rule Number 6 – Don't Pass on Snacks

It is important to eat enough of the right foods to keep you blood glucose levels steady throughout the day, and that will keep your energy levels steady as well. Snack on dried fruit and nuts, yoghurt with granola, whole grain crackers, fresh raw vegetables and fruits.

Rule Number 7 – Drink Your Fluids

Hydration is an important part of weight loss and of keeping your energy levels high. Your body needs a lot of water to function at its best but, unless you are doing endurance training, skip the energy drinks and vitamin waters. Instead, drink plain water or water with fresh fruit chunks in it and aim to drink at least one cup every couple of hours.

Rule Number 8 – Be a Designated Driver

That will help you to cut out one of the biggest enemies of those who want to lose weight – alcohol. As well as acting as a depressant, alcohol can also act as a stimulant, interrupting your sleep patterns and causing tiredness the following day. If you are relying on a drink every night to help you fall asleep, you are doing the wrong thing. Cutting out the alcohol will help you to sleep better.

If you do want to have a drink occasionally, stick to red wine. It is an antioxidant but do be aware that you cannot drink if you are on certain medications, have high blood pressure or anxiety.

Rule Number 9 – Caffeine – Little or None

Caffeine should be used carefully and in small amounts. Although it seems as if it is giving you an energy boost, it won't last for long and you will know it when it wears off. And never use caffeine as a meal replacement! Green tea is a better choice of caffeine as it also contains antioxidants and theanine, which is an essential amino acid that helps you to stay calm.

Rule Number 10 – Eat Power Foods

Try to stick to nutritional foods that provide energy, a list of 10 are below. Later on I will go into more details on foods to eat to help you burn off fat.

- Nuts, especially almonds
- Avocado
- Dark leafy greens, such as watercress, kale, spinach, collard or beet greens
- Whole grains that are intact, like quinoa, millet, brown rice or amaranth

- Ground flax seeds
- White beans, lentils, black beans
- Dried fruits such as dates but in moderation
- Berries – blackberries, strawberries, raspberries, blueberries, etc.
- Sea vegetables such as Nori, hijiki, dulse, etc.
- Edamame – whole young soy beans

Nicholas Bjorn

Chapter 2 – Top 10 Herbs and Spices to Help Improve Health and Weight Loss

Herbs and spices are a fantastic way of giving otherwise bland food a taste boost and using them is one of the best ways to enjoy nutritious foods that may not taste so great. Not many people know that herbs and spices are full of health benefits. The following are ten of the best to boost your health and excite your taste buds.

Cayenne Pepper

Adds a dash of spice and also helps to enhance bodily functions. Cayenne helps to boost the metabolism, in turn increasing the amount of fat that your body burns off and it improves your blood flow. This means that the essential nutrients and vitamins in your food are moved through the body far more efficiently, allowing your body to function better.

Black Pepper

Similar to cayenne, black pepper helps to boost the metabolism and it helps to improve the digestive process, which in turn helps the body to shed weight. It also contains anti-cancer properties.

Ginger

Ginger is good for suppressing the appetite and aiding digestion. It also works to warm up the body, increasing metabolism and helping more calories to burn off. Ginger is good for shifting toxins out of the body, in particular out of the fat cells.

Ginseng

Ginseng helps to boost metabolism and raise energy levels and is popular in energy drinks. It is a great one to use just before you do short high intensity workouts.

Chamomile Tea

Chamomile tea is great for relaxation and helps to reduce stress levels. It also helps to stop emotional eating in the evenings, thus preventing weight gain and it helps you to sleep better. Chamomile contains anti-inflammatory properties, helping to reduce the inflammation that causes so many different diseases, and it is high in antioxidants, eliminating free radicals from the body.

Cumin

Cumin tends to be mixed with other spices to give a nice flavor to Mexican, Indian, Middle Eastern and Mediterranean foods. It is used as a part of Ayurvedic medicine, helps to boost your immune system, decrease your cholesterol and contains anti-oxidant properties. It helps to increase the energy levels, allowing for more calories to be burned off.

Turmeric

Turmeric is fantastic for people who crave junk food. It helps to boost the function of the liver and to balance out hormones, which also prevents binges. It is a powerful antioxidant that helps to maintain good joints and skin, as well as vision. It works to enhance the immune system, digestive processes and the function of the liver as well as stabilizing blood glucose levels and cutting down on the amount of fat storage.

Cinnamon

This is a sweet spice that helps to boost metabolism and improve insulin sensitivity, thus helping to boost fat burning and control the blood sugar levels.

Mustard

Mustard helps to boost weight loss because it is full of B-complex vitamins, such as niacin, folates, riboflavin and thiamine, all of which increase the metabolism. One teaspoon of mustard can help to boost metabolism by 25%. Mustard is also high in magnesium and selenium which provides anti-inflammatory properties to help fight off disease. It is also a good source of zeaxanthins, carotenes and luteins, all of which are good antioxidants that help to eliminate free radicals.

Cardamom

This is a sweet spice that is used in Indian cooking and it helps to promote a healthy digestion and increases your metabolism. It is a commonly used ingredient in Ayurvedic medicine and has been shown to help mouth ulcers, high blood pressure, and depression. It has both anti-oxidative and anti-inflammatory properties and can also help to slow down the aging process.

So, the next time you are preparing your meals, add in one or more of these herbs and spices. Not only will your food taste nicer, your health will be better and your metabolism will be faster, helping you to burn off fat more efficiently.

Chapter 3 – 36 Fat Burning Super Foods

Food is not our enemy but so many diets will have you believe that it is. You don't need to eat a diet that is lacking in taste or looks to lose weight and you certainly do not need to deprive yourself just because the latest fad diet says you mustn't at certain foods. The following 36 foods are super foods that will help you to burn off fat more efficiently. However, don't get stuck on just one of them; introduce a few of them at a time to your weekly menu and, as time goes on, you will find that you are eating more and more of them.

Tomatoes

Who really cares if a tomato is a fruit or a vegetable? All that is important is knowing that a tomato contains loads of goodness that can help your body in the long terms and, over the short term, it can help you to lose some weight. They are low in calories but contain enough fiber to keep you regular and make you feel fuller. Tomatoes contain lycopene as well, which are antioxidants, helpful in removing free radicals and other toxins from your system.

Oranges

Oranges are full of vitamin C, which is needed to keep your body functioning at an optimal level. However, many people avoid oranges when they are trying to burn fat because they are worried about the sugar level. Oranges do contain sugar and, if you eat too many of them and don't burn off the sugar, it can turn to fat. However, they are low in calories and high in fiber, which helps keep your glucose levels regular. To help you to lose weight, moderate how much you eat and use it as a way of curbing a craving for candy.

Oats

Oats contain fiber, which helps to boost the metabolism, although many of those who do diets like Atkins and Paleo would disagree. A bowl of oatmeal is a fabulous way to start off the day. It isn't just full of fiber; it also contains anti-oxidants and lots of other minerals. Oats are a good way of cutting cholesterol levels.

Spices

You do not need to eat bland tasteless food when you are trying to shed some pounds so get experimenting with the contents of your spice rack. Some of them contain thermo genic properties, which help to boost the metabolism, and all of them give dishes a great taste. Mustard seed goes great on an entrée and will boost your metabolism while ginger helps your digestive system. Ginseng boosts energy and black pepper can help you to burn off calories. Turmeric is good for breaking up fat.

Sweet Potatoes

These are a fantastic addition to a diet, as a replacement for normal potatoes because they contain fewer calories and can help you to feel fuller for longer. Sweet potatoes are also loaded with potassium, fiber, vitamin B6 and vitamin C, making them the perfect replacement for a food that is normally shunned by dieters everywhere.

Apples

Not many people realize just how good an apple is. They are sweet enough to be a good replacement for sweet cravings and you can easily see why they end up in desserts. They are also low in calories, low in fat and low in sodium while being high in fiber. The fiber fills you up for longer and stops you from eating in between meals, and they also help with your digestive system too. Make sure you chew and apple thoroughly to get the best out of it.

Nuts

Every diet plan in the world include nuts and they are the one food that unites the vegetarians with the meat loving paleo dieters. They come straight from the earth and a small handful of nuts, raw and organic ones like pecans, walnuts or almonds, can be a tasty and filling snack that keep soya going for a few hours. You can also chop them and add them to a salad or sprinkle them over your food. Nuts are full of good healthy fats and full of flavor.

Quinoa

Quinoa is just starting to become popular in mainstream diets and the weight loss normally happens when you switch out rice or potatoes, or other starchy sides with quinoa. You get the full benefits of a well-rounded meals with all the vitamins contained in the quinoa. It is low in calories, low GI and full of taste.

Beans

Beans are a staple part of many diets and should be included as part of your weekly menu. They help to regulate glucose levels, help with digestion because of their high fiber content and are a great replacement for high carb foods. Black beans are particularly good for snacking on and you will find that many restaurants provide them as an alternative to bread.

Egg Whites

The egg debate is an age-old one. Some people say the yolks are fine to eat, others say they are not okay to eat and that you should only eat egg whites. Whole eggs are a fantastic source of protein and the biggest debate rages around the cholesterol and fat levels in the yolks. If you want to be safe, eat the whites on and start adding yolks back in at a later date.

Grapefruit

Grapefruits are an excellent fat burning food and this is being proved with more research every year. Grapefruit helps to kick start the digestive system, making fat burning an easier and more efficient process. You can start with pure grapefruit juice if you want and work your way up to eating a grapefruit.

Chicken Breast

Chicken breast is a staple part of many diets, although it is obviously no good if you are going vegetarian or vegan. It is low in fat and high in protein and is far healthier to eat than the dark meat from a chicken. Do remember to take the skin off, as this is where all the fat is and use a variety of spices and herbs to boost the flavor. Combine eating chicken breast with strength training to help tone up your muscles, which will boost your metabolism rate as well.

Bananas

Bananas are one of the most natural foods to eat and are the subject of many research programs for their effect on weight loss. They are so easy to add in to your diet on a daily basis because they are such a versatile fruit. They can be eaten on their own, chopped up and added to oatmeal or yoghurt and are a great source of potassium, natural sugar and energy.

Pears

Pears are often dismissed from a diet but they really should be included. They are full of flavor, and contain a whole range of benefits, which are great for weight loss. They help you to feel fuller for longer and they are different in consistency to apples and other fruits, which makes their fiber content more effective than others are. They can be eaten as they are, chopped up or cooked.

Pine Nuts

Pine nuts include a phytonutrient that can help to suppress the appetite, which means you can ditch the cost of buying expensive diet pills that are full of chemicals to do the same thing. They are tiny and they are crunchy so you can eat a lot without worrying about the effect of them and without ruining your weight loss efforts. These are one food you can binge on without any trouble.

Mushrooms

You won't see the benefits if you switch pepperoni for mushrooms on your next pizza but if you start increasing the amount you are eating, along with a range of other healthier foods, you will see a difference, because they are low in calories and high in vitamins. Don't be boring though; try all different ones from the supermarket and enjoy a range of textures, flavors and other great benefits.

Lentils

Lentils are another food that is gaining in popularity and are not just for a vegetarian diet. They contain fiber, which helps your digestive system keep your blood sugar from spiking and help you to feel fuller for longer. They are also full of protein and help to keep cholesterol levels down as well as helping the body to process carbohydrates better.

Hot Peppers

Jalapenos, chipotles and habaneros peppers are excellent weight loss foods while adding a healthy kick to the flavor of a dish. Instead of ruining your stomach lining like some believe, these will actually help to protect your stomach and prevent ulcers by killing off the bad bacteria.

Broccoli

Broccoli is one of the best superfoods. Not only are they full of anti-oxidants, they are also jam packed with nutrients and fiber. They fill you up quickly and keep your digestive system clear which makes you feel so much better. Add spices or peppers to it to give it more flavor. Broccoli with a sprinkling of turmeric has been proven to keep prostate cancer at bay as well as help you lose weight.

Organic Lean Meats

Lean meats contain all of the protein you need without the fat levels but, if you are looking to lose weight, go for organic meats. With normal meats, the animals are pumped full of growth hormones, antibiotics and other nasty things which all end up in what you get on your plate and can slow down your weight loss. Organic meat do not contain any more nutrients than normal meat but this is a case of what it doesn't contain that makes it better. If organic is not n supply, look for grass-fed or all-natural brands.

Cantaloupe Melon

There are those who say that eating a cantaloupe burns off more calories than it contains but that is still up for debate. Whatever the outcome, it is a great food for helping to lose weight because, while it is sweet, it is low in calories, contains fiber and helps keep you moving. It is good on its own, in a fruit salad or even in a smoothie with other fruits and vegetables. Cantaloupe melon can also help to keep your skin looking great.

Spinach

Spinach is so often left lying on the plate but it is a fantastic food for health and weight loss. It is full of antioxidants, vitamins and minerals and is good to eat in a number of ways. Cook it, eat it raw in a salad, however you want. It adds bulk without adding calories. Try to go for organic and buy in bulk if you buy fresh because you can freeze it for a later date.

Green Tea

Green tea is full of antioxidants and can help you to burn off fat. This is because green tea contains catechins, which help your body to start burning off more calories and well as fat. It isn't processed like so many other teas, and is packed with antioxidants and phytonutrients that make it one of the superstar super foods.

Cinnamon

Cinnamon is one of the most powerful spices and is no longer just used for cooking. Instead, you can get the benefits from cinnamon by adding a teaspoon a day into your diet. It works by regulating your blood sugar levels, which also plays a big part in the way you are feeling throughout the day. Low blood sugar levels are indicated by a sluggish heavy feeling. Keeping your sugar levels even can also help to stop cravings. One good way is to have a drink of honey and cinnamon in hot water every day.

Asparagus

Asparagus plays a big role in weight loss with lots of different benefits and each benefit plays a specific role in weight loss. Asparagus helps to eliminate toxins from the body, helps with the digestion process and leaves the good bacteria thriving in your gut. It also has loads of vitamins, minerals and antioxidants. It tastes nice and can also be boosted with spices and seasonings.

Avocado

Avocado is a great slimming aid and contain loads of healthy fats. They were avoided for a long time because of that fat content, at a time when fat was given the label of being evil but we now know that not all fats are bad and that god fats can help to burn fat. Add avocado to salads, sandwiches, eat them as they are or make your own guacamole with them.

Peanut Butter

Peanut butter contains good fats that help to burn fat but do go for organic peanut butter as it doesn't contain any of them extra salt and sugar and tat standard peanut butter contains. It can be eaten as part of a smoothie or a piece of celery dipped in peanut butter makes a great filling snack. You can also have almond butter but it is more expensive.

Salmon

Salmon, like other fish, contains a high level of omega 3 and this is one thing that is sorely lacking in many diets today. It may be classed as a fatty fish but it is not high in saturated fats, which are the bad fats and the omega 3 content makes it better than anything else. You would need to add this in gradually to see how your body takes to it so start with once a week. If you get on with it, increase that and look around for some great tasting salmon recipes.

Apple Cider Vinegar

Go for raw organic apple cider vinegar because it contains enzymes that help your digestive system and can help with weight loss over time. The recommended way is to add it to filtered or distilled water and drink it before you eat; this helps your food to be properly digested so that your body gets all the goodness from the nutrients instead of wasting them. It can also help suppress the appetite so drink it if you find yourself hungry between meals.

Greek Yoghurt

Greek yoghurt is healthier than any other yoghurt because it is full of proteins and has a lower sugar content than normal yoghurt. You don't have to use it as a substitute for normal yoghurt though; you can use it in place of sour cream, cutting down fat and calories and you can also experiment with baking, using it in place of other fats and oils. This could take a bit of trial and error to get it right though.

Olive Oil

Olive oil is a much healthier oil than vegetable or seed oils and it can be used in a variety of ways. Not only can you add it to salads, either on its own or as part of a salad dressing, you can also use it for cooking in.

Blueberries

Blueberries are excellent for fat loss, not just weight. They help to break down sugars and fats in the body as well as tasting amazing. You can use them to add flavor to any meal and they also go well with other fruits – just skip the cream and sugar! Add them to yoghurt or oatmeal for a tasty breakfast or snack.

Turkey Breast

Turkey breast is good for those moments when you are hungry and feel as though you are going to cave in. It is a good source of lean protein and is popular on low or no carb diets. It is a god meat to eat if you are strength training and building up muscle, as well as being able to boost your metabolism.

Flax Seeds

Flax seed can be sprinkled on just about anything you want and it is a better option than sugar. It contains healthy doses of fiber, omega 3 and helps to keep you feeling fuller for longer. The essential fatty acids contained in flax seed helps to boost metabolism and lower bad cholesterol levels.

Use Fresh and Organic

Use fresh ingredients wherever possible and stick to organic. Processed foods are lower in antioxidants and have little weight loss power left in them. Organic foods are best because they don't contain the chemicals and have not been genetically modified.

You can make soups and smoothies out of some of the ingredients on this list and this is a great way to get the benefits without eating a plate of raw food. Soup is excellent for weight loss and is helps with the digestion process and you can put lots of different foods together in the same soup for a real fat busting meal that is packed full of vitamins. You can have the soup as a starter or as a meal on its own. It is also much easier to digest than some foods.

Chapter 4 - The Top 20 Superfoods You Should be Eating

Everyone wants to be healthy and fit. There are many ways to stay healthy and fit, but all of them circle back to two things: exercise and diet. Nowadays, people find it difficult to follow a diet routine and an exercise regime. But if you want to stay healthy, there are no alternatives to these two options. Almost every day, we are introduced to a new form of exercise or diet routine. One such new (but really old) introduction to the world of diet is 'superfoods.'

Superfoods have become really popular nowadays thanks to the publicity they have received in recent times. There are many types of superfoods, most of them being plant-based, but there are also many superfoods that are dairy or fish-based. All these foods contain high amounts of nutrients. Some commonly found superfoods include salmon, kale, apples, blueberries, etc.

There exists no specific definition of superfoods. They are not a separate food group. Rather, superfoods are foods that contain high amounts of nutrients and are generally good for the health of your heart. Most of the superfoods contain a variety of nutrients, including protein, fats, vitamins, and essential minerals. They also contain many different antioxidants, which make them effective against cancer and similar diseases.

Many superfoods also contain a high amount of healthy fats, which are great for the health of your heart. They are also good for the health of your cardiovascular system. Many superfoods are also effective against digestive problems as well. They contain high amounts of phytochemicals that have many health benefits. Phytochemicals provide foods their deep color and taste. Adding superfoods to your day-to-day diet can help you a lot. It can bring in a lot of positive changes in your lifestyle. It can help you become fit and healthy.

In this chapter, let us have a look at twenty important superfoods that you can incorporate into your daily meals. Almost all of these superfoods are easily available on the market. Most of them are quite affordable. They are also versatile, and you can make a variety of recipes with them.

Broccoli

Broccoli is considered to be one of the healthiest vegetables as it is packed with nutrients. It contains a high amount of fiber and is rich in antioxidants as well. These properties of broccoli allow it to fight cancer. Its high antioxidant content is good for the repair of body cells and tissues. It also contains high amounts of minerals and vitamins. Broccoli is also great for the cardiovascular system and immune system. It has anti-inflammatory properties, which makes it an overall healthy vegetable. Along with its high fiber content, it is low in fats, which makes it best for people who are trying to lose weight.

Broccoli, along with other cruciferous vegetables, can reduce the growth of cancer cells. Broccoli can also reduce the blood sugar levels and is thus a boon for diabetics. Broccoli can also prevent (and reduce) cardiovascular tissue damage.

As said above, broccoli contains a high amount of fiber, which is great for digestive health. It makes bowel movements regular and smooth. Dark green vegetables such as broccoli contain a lot of nutrients that can prevent the signs of aging. One such nutrient is sulforaphane. Sulforaphane is also good for the health of the brain.

Broccoli contains a high amount of vitamin C. Vitamin C is good for the immune system. It is also good for oral health and can keep your teeth healthy. Broccoli is also good for your bones as it contains high amounts of phosphorous, calcium, and vitamin K. According to some studies, broccoli can even control joint disorders.

Broccoli is a highly recommended food for pregnant or lactating women. Broccoli is rich in nutrients, which ensures the healthy development of the fetus. It helps lactating women stay healthy. It is high in folate, which is great for the health of new mothers.

Broccoli can also control inflammation and boost immune power. It can also regulate blood sugar levels. Thus it is clear that broccoli is a superfood that can help you get healthy and fit. There are various ways of consuming broccoli. To avoid repetition, use different methods every time you cook broccoli.

Avocado

Avocado is a green, pear-shaped fruit that is often referred to as an "alligator pear." It is prized for its healthy fats, fiber, and various important nutrients. There are many types of avocado that vary in shape and color — from pear-shaped to round and green to black.

Avocados have become a highly popular food and ingredient today. They are consumed in a variety of forms and are often the main ingredient in salads, dips, shakes, etc. They are rich in vitamins- especially vitamin B, potassium, and folic acid. Another aspect that makes avocados great for health is that it allows the body to absorb nutrients effectively. This means that avocados help you to absorb the nutrients provided by other food in a more efficient manner. This is especially true in the case of carotenoids, which is an essential cancer-fighting compound.

Avocados contain high amounts of monounsaturated fatty acids, such as oleic acids. This allows them to control and manage cholesterol levels. Oleic acid is also good for preventing breast cancer.

Avocados are full of potassium, which is good for the health of the heart and bones. It can prevent many heart diseases and disorders and can also prevent stroke. It is also good for digestion and is often used for 'detox' process. Along with potassium, avocados also contain high amounts of vitamin C, B6, and D, along with manganese, and riboflavin. All these components work together to improve your immune system. They are also a good source of vitamins A and E, which can prevent cancer to a certain extent.

Another aspect that makes avocados great is that they are rich in omega-3. It reduces the risk of heart diseases and disorder and is good for your arteries. They also contain high amounts of lecithin, a type of fatty acid that is crucial for healthy nervous tissues.

Avocados are full of fiber as well. Fiber is essential for digestive health, and it can also help you lose weight. Fiber satiates you and thus prevents you from eating unnecessary and empty calories. According to various surveys, people who eat avocados regularly are comparatively healthier than those who don't. They also have a lower risk of developing metabolic diseases. Avocados contain high amounts of lutein and zeaxanthin. These antioxidants are good for the health of your eyes and optic nerves. They can also help you prevent cataract and macular degeneration.

Avocados are great for people who want to lose weight. It can help you keep full for a long time. Avocados are low in carbs and thus can help you lose weight efficiently. Incorporating avocados in your daily diet is easy as it is tasty and easy to use. You can use avocados in various forms, including avocado butter, shakes, salad, toast, etc.

Sweet Potato

Sweet potato is a delicious and nutrient-rich vegetable that is known for its distinctive sweet flavor. It is a highly versatile and healthful vegetable that is readily available in the market. Although people confuse sweet potato with yam all the time, both of them are different. Sweet potato is one of the most easily available and nutrient-rich superfoods. It contains high amounts of beta-carotene, which is a great antioxidant.

Sweet potato also contains high amounts of vitamin A. This vitamin is essential for the health of our bones, skin, immune system, eyes, and reproductive system as well. Sweet potato also has nutrients that can help you prevent cancer. It also contains high amounts of vitamin C, which is great for people who have asthma or arthritis. It can also help people who have diabetes as it has a very low glycemic index, which means it does not have a significant effect on blood glucose levels.

As said above, sweet potato is sweet in taste and is a starchy root vegetable that is grown all around the globe. This tube is available in various sizes, shapes, and colors. They contain high amounts of fiber, which makes them a great food for people who are trying to lose weight. They also increase the number of good gut bacteria that is good for the digestive system.

Sweet potatoes contain high amounts of different antioxidants. These antioxidants are helpful against various types of cancers. For instance, sweet potato contains anthocyanin, an antioxidant that is well known for slowing down the growth of cancerous cells of cancers affecting bladder, colon, breast, and the stomach. Sweet potatoes are also a rich source of beta-carotene, which is good for optical health.

Sweet potatoes are extremely versatile and can be used like regular potatoes. There are many different ways of cooking sweet potatoes. They can be boiled, roasted, baked, fried pan-cooked, or steamed. It is possible to consume them with skin or without skin as well. If you like eating chips, try eating sweet potato chips. These chips are healthier than regular chips. As sweet potatoes are naturally sweet, they go well with many different flavors. You can make sweet as well as savory dishes with sweet potatoes.

Wheat Grass

Wheatgrass is a superfood made out of the Triticum Aestivum plant. It contains high amounts of nutrients that are great for your health. It is generally consumed in the form of fresh juice, but nowadays, it is also available in the form of powder. The powder is far more convenient than the juice. While a lot of people now understand the importance of wheatgrass, many people are still unaware of its benefits, which is why it still remains an underrated superfood. If consumed daily, wheatgrass can help you tackle many diseases and disorders.

As said above, wheatgrass is full of a variety of nutrients that are necessary for our body. Wheatgrass also has many nourishing and therapeutic properties. It contains many different vitamins and minerals that keep fit and active. It also contains a variety of enzymes that are good for your digestive system. Another factor that makes wheatgrass really great is that it improves and enhances the immune system. It is also good for people who are trying to lose weight because it tackles cholesterol levels and minimizes them. Wheatgrass also makes you calm and relaxed. It can relieve you of anxiety. It improves mental function. It reduces stress. It improves cognitive function and can also be used to prevent the symptoms of Alzheimer's disease.

Salmon

Salmon is a highly nutritious fish that is considered to be an important superfood. It contains high amounts of omega three and healthy fats. The nutrients and oil present in salmon are rarely found in other species of fish, which makes salmon one of the healthiest fish. Salmon contains a high amount of polyunsaturated fats. These fats reduce the levels of serum triglycerides and can enhance brain functioning and cardiovascular health as well.

It is true that salmon is a pricey seafood option, but the number of nutrients (and taste) present in it makes it worth it. It considered being the best source of dietary omega 3. Other, considerably cost-effective fish such as herring roe and sardines too contain omega-3, but salmon contain the highest amounts.

Fish is a really good source of omega 3 as they provide long-chain polyunsaturated fatty acids. These acids are as follows: Eicosapentacnoic and docosahexaenoic acid (EPA and DHA). Such combinations are only found in seafood and marine algae or seaweed. Terrain plants provide short-chain omega-3 alpha-linolenic acid (ALA). The human body can utilize ALA to synthesize EPA and DHA, but getting them directly from the source is always better as it reduces the work and energy required. For instance, one 4 oz portion of cooked salmon can provide approximately 2000 mg of omega-3s.

The human body needs L-tryptophan (an amino acid) to make melatonin. This acid is found in abundance in salmon. This is why people who eat salmon regularly rarely face any sleep-related problems. A 4 oz serving of salmon contains approximately 250–400 mg of L-tryptophan.

The vitamin B family is necessary for the body as these vitamins are used to regulate energy metabolism and enhance tissue formation as well. Salmon contains a lot of vitamin Bs, including B2, B3, B6, and B12. If you are a pescatarian, then eating salmon is one of the best ways to get vitamin B12. A 4 oz piece of salmon contains 5.7 mcg of B12 or 236% of the recommended daily intake.

Salmon also contains high amounts of minerals, such as phosphorus and calcium. These minerals are good for the health of your teeth and bones. It also contains other trace materials such as selenium, which is a great antioxidant. A 4 oz serving of salmon provides 365 mg of phosphorus or 52% of the recommended daily intake.

Salmon is also a great source of protein. Salmon contains various amino acids that are essential for the health of your body. It also contains proteins such as calcitonin, which promotes healthy joints and bones.

Astaxanthin is another antioxidant that is found in abundance in salmon and similar seafood. It is a fat-soluble pigment that is red in color; this is why salmon looks so red. It also contains high amounts of carotenoids that can reduce the number of free radicals. This is why salmon is considered to be one of the best superfoods.

Pomegranate Seeds

Pomegranate is considered to be one of the best superfoods currently available. It has been used since ancient times in the Middle East and has been celebrated for its taste and health benefits. The outer skin of the pomegranate is tough, but the insides are juicy, delicious, and blood red.

The seeds of pomegranate are slightly tart and sweet. These seeds not only help you stay healthy but also free of disease. They are a great addition to your salads as they will not only make it more colorful and healthy, but it will make your salads tasty as well.

As said earlier, pomegranates were used in Asia, India, Africa, and the Mediterranean since ancient times. In ancient times, pomegranates were used to denote fertility. It is one of the most represented fruits in art throughout the centuries.

Pomegranate was introduced to North America around a few centuries ago. It is now grown in abundance in parts of Arizona and California. All the parts of pomegranates contain immense amounts of nutrients. This is why pomegranates have become such a rage in the world of superfoods. Nowadays, pomegranates are easily available in the market in the form of juices, extracts, powders, supplements, etc. The fruits are available in abundance in supermarkets.

Pomegranates can help you lower cholesterol, which makes them great for cardiovascular and heart diseases. Pomegranates also contain high amounts of vitamin C, which provides them immense anti-inflammatory properties. Pomegranates are also potent against certain cancers and Type 2 diabetes as well. Pomegranates also contain high amounts of antioxidants, which can help to reduce high blood pressure. Pomegranate is also good for the health of your brain, arteries, and heart.

According to certain studies, if you consume around 8 oz of pomegranate juice daily, it can work wonders for your health. Pomegranate is also good for 'masculine health.' It can improve erections and can also slow down the growth of prostate cancer cells as well.

Blueberries

Blueberries are versatile fruits that can be either eaten raw and fresh or can be utilized in a variety of recipes as well. Blueberries can be used fresh or can be eaten frozen as well.

Blueberries contain high amounts of anthocyanin. This compound gives them a distinct color. It is also responsible for its numerous health benefits. Blueberries are good for the health of your heart. They are also good for your skin, hair, blood pressure, bone strength, diabetes, mental health, and cancer. One cup of blueberries can provide you with 24% of the daily total vitamin C requirement.

As said above, blueberries are exceptionally versatile, and they can be used in a variety of forms and in a variety of recipes as well. For instance, blueberries are often used to top salads, ice cream, yogurt, shakes, pancakes, cereals, oatmeal, and salads too. They can also be blended into syrups and smoothies. You can also add them to sweetbreads and muffins. You can make a variety of desserts with blueberries.

Blueberries also contain high amounts of vitamin K. This is why people who are on blood thinners should avoid using a lot of blueberries or should consult their health professional before eating a lot of blueberries.

Blueberries contain many different flavonoids. Flavonoids are antioxidants that have multiple health benefits.

Eating a variety of fruits and vegetables is one of the best ways to stay healthy and tackle diseases and disorders. For instance, a lot of studies have proved the consuming blueberries can help you tackle obesity, heart problems, diabetes, and various other diseases as well. Blueberries can improve your overall health. Blueberries are also good for people who are trying to lose weight. They are also good for the health of your skin and hair.

Blueberries are often sold frozen. While freezing them ensures a long shelf life, the process removes many essential nutrients. According to a study, the amount of anthocyanin in frozen blueberries decreases rapidly, and in a couple of months, it can go down by 30-40 %. More research is required regarding this. But it is always better to buy and eat fresh blueberries whenever you can. Try to find organic berries.

Blueberries contain a variety of minerals as well. For instance, they are rich in calcium, phosphorus, iron, magnesium, zinc, manganese, and vitamin K. All these nutrients are good for the health of your bones. If you consume adequate amounts of vitamins and minerals, your bones become healthy and non-brittle. Iron and zinc are responsible for the health of your joints. Vitamin K deficiency often leads to brittle bones. This is because vitamin K improves the absorption of calcium. A low amount of vitamin K ultimately leads to a low amount of calcium.

Collagen is essential for the health of our skin. It keeps it tight, young, fresh, and healthy. Collagen needs a lot of vitamin C to perform properly. Collagen also protects the skin from various damaging factors such as pollution, the sun, and smoke. Blueberries contain high amounts of vitamin C, which enhances the potency of collagen. Thus, blueberries can help you achieve beautiful and attractive looking skin.

Blueberries contain no sodium. Excessive sodium is bad for your health, especially for your blood pressure. On the other hand, blueberries are full of calcium, potassium, and magnesium. The deficiency of these minerals can often lead to high blood pressure. Thus, blueberries can help you regulate your blood pressure.

A high fiber diet is recommended for people who have Type 1 diabetes. A high fiber diet can help to lower blood glucose levels. Similarly, people suffering from Type 2 diabetes can also benefit a lot from consuming a high fiber diet. A single cup of blueberries contains around 3.6 grams of fiber.

Blueberries are also good for the health of your heart. They contain high amounts of potassium, fiber, folate, vitamin B6, vitamin C, and phytonutrients. All these nutrients are essential for the health of your heart. Blueberries contain no cholesterol. The fiber in blueberries can reduce the amount of cholesterol present in the body already.

Homocysteine is a harmful chemical that is present in our body. A lot of homocysteine can lead to clogging and damaging blood vessels. It is extremely dangerous for the health of or heart. Blueberries contain a high amount of vitamin B6 and folate, which can prevent the buildup of homocysteine.

According to a study, it was found that women who consumed around three servings of blueberries every week showed a reduced risk of heart diseases and disorders. The various vitamins present in blueberries act as antioxidants that can tackle free radicals present in the body.

According to research, antioxidants can also prevent the growth of tumors and reduce inflammation. They can slow down the growth of cancer cells in the lungs, esophagus, mouth, pharynx, pancreas, colon, and prostate. They can also prevent endometrial cancer, as well.

Blueberries are rich in folate. Folate plays a crucial role in the repair and synthesis of DNA. Due to this, the DNA does not mutate. DNA mutations are often responsible for cancer.

Blueberries can also tackle cognitive damage, especially in women. Similar studies have proved how blueberries can improve memory and coordination. It can also help to prevent and tackle other brain-related problems.

Blueberries are also great against constipation. They are good for the health of your digestive system. They contain lots of fiber, which is good for digestion. Dietary fiber is also good for weight loss and weight management. High fiber foods lead to early satiation. This way, you do not end up consuming a lot of empty calories, making blueberries a miracle berry!

Quinoa

Quinoa has become a rage in the world of fitness and health now. Quinoa is considered one of the healthiest and nutrient-rich foods available in the market. It is a highly healthy and delicious food. It is a highly versatile and incredible food that is a great source of carbs. Many people believe that quinoa is a grain just like rice or wheat, but it is quite different than them. In fact, quinoa is not a grain at all. It is known as pseudo-grain. It is a form of seed that is highly nutritious.

Quinoa is one of the most nutrient-dense carbs available today. It has around six grams of proteins per cup. It is also the only carb source that contains all nine essential amino acids. Along with this, quinoa is a complete protein. It also contains a high amount of lysine. Lysine is an amino acid that is necessary for healing and repairing muscles. This is why many gym rats generally include quinoa in their diet.

Quinoa also has many other benefits, such as it is full of various minerals and vitamins. It is a rich source of copper, iron, phosphorus, and manganese. Manganese and copper control free radicals and are good for the health of bones and teeth. Phosphorous and iron play an integral role in the creation of energy. Then it can also help against the development of cancer cells. Another point that makes quinoa really great is that it is full of fiber. Each serving contains around 2.5 grams of fiber. Fiber is great for people who are trying to lose weight. It satiates you and keeps you feeling full for a long time. This way, you do not consume random, useless calories. Fiber is also good for the health of your digestive tract. It is also good for diabetics as it improves the function of insulin.

Nowadays, there are many different recipes of quinoa available online. While North America is trying to grow quinoa locally, a lot of quinoa is still imported from South America. Due to the increasing demands of quinoa, it has become a priced commodity. But the price is definitely worth the health benefits of the product. This is why people are still buying quinoa in abundance.

Nowadays, quinoa is available in a variety of forms. For instance, you can now buy quinoa cereal, pasta, flour, cookies, etc. It is an extremely versatile food product and can be used in a variety of recipes. You can make delicious desserts, cookies, granola bars, cakes, side dishes, breakfast foods, shakes, etc. from quinoa. It is easy to use, which is why many people now try to incorporate it into their daily meals.

Quinoa is a boon for people who are allergic to gluten. It contains no gluten and is thus great for people who are on a no-gluten diet. Gluten is found in many essential grains such as rye, oats, wheat, and barley, which make them unsuitable for anyone who has celiac disease or is allergic to gluten. Quinoa is rich in nutrients and contains no gluten, which has made it really popular with the gluten-free community.

Quinoa has a slightly nutty flavor that is not at all overpowering and goes well with almost everything. It is easy to cook, and it hardly takes more than 12-15 minutes to get done. It is also popular with kids in the form of cereal and cookies.

Almonds

Almonds are not only tasty, but they are also full of nutrients. They contain high amounts of minerals, proteins, vitamins, fiber, etc. Their nutrition makes them a really healthy superfood. For instance, only a handful of almonds contain around 1/8th of our daily protein needs. Almonds are versatile, and there are multiple ways to eat them. You can eat them raw, or you can also toast them. They are often added to sweet as well as savory dishes as toppings or garnish. They are a great addition to salads as they provide a good crunch to it. Nowadays, almonds are available in a variety of forms, including chopped almonds, peeled almonds, slivered almonds, sliced almonds, almond flakes, almond flour, almond oil, almond milk, and almond butter. Almond is known as a nut, but it is actually a seed full of nutrients.

Almond trees are one of the earliest plants that human beings cultivated. Archaeologists have found evidence showcasing that people in Jordan domesticated almond trees around 5000 years ago. Almonds are full of fats, but they are full of unsaturated fats. Unsaturated fats are healthy and essential for the body. They do not increase LDL or low-density lipoprotein. LDL is often known as "bad" cholesterol.

According to the AHA or American Heart Association, moderate amounts of unsaturated fats can improve your cholesterol levels. Almonds contain no cholesterol. According to a study published in 2005 says that almonds also contain high amounts of vitamin E. Vitamin E is an essential antioxidant that can stop the oxidization process that is responsible for the clogging of arteries. Along with this, another study conducted in 2018 found the same results. According to this study, almonds can help to increase or maintain the levels of HDL or high-density lipoprotein or "good" cholesterol. According to this study, people are recommended to consume at least 45 grams of almonds a day for cardiovascular health.

According to a 2015 study, almonds can help against cancer as well. The study says that almonds can reduce the risk of breast cancer by about two to three times. Peanuts and walnuts, too, were found to be helpful against breast cancer.

In another study conducted in 2011, around 20 people suffering from Type 2 diabetes were observed. They were asked to eat 60 g of almonds every day for 12 weeks. It was found that the almonds improved their blood lipids, blood sugar levels, and fat levels as well.

One oz of almonds contains around 76. 5 mg of magnesium on average. This is around 20-24% of the total daily requirement of a healthy adult. While magnesium supplements are a great way to tackle deficiency, healthy people can eat almonds to avoid becoming deficient.

Almonds contain high amounts of fibers, proteins, and healthy fats. They are low in carbs. These factors make them great for people who are trying to lose weight. According to a study conducted in 2015, people who eat almonds as morning snacks eat fewer calories throughout the day. This is because almonds contain fiber, which helps you stay satiated for a long time. This is why almonds are often a staple ingredient of breakfast cereals and muesli.

Almonds are also a rich source of vitamin K, manganese, calcium, copper, zinc, and protein. All these are responsible for good and healthy bones.

Beet Roots

Beetroot is a delicious, healthy, and great looking vegetable that is packed with nutrients. Beet leaves are healthy as well. Beetroot has been used since ancient times for various medical purposes. For instance, it was once upon a time used to treat fevers, skin issues, constipation, etc.

Beetroot contains high amounts of folate and iron. Folate is naturally occurring folic acid, which is good for your health. It also contains high amounts of magnesium, nitrates, betaine, betacyanin, and many other antioxidants that are good for health. According to recent studies, it has been proven that beetroots can also help to lower blood pressure and can prevent dementia as well. It is great for gym rats as it increases stamina.

As said above, beetroot contains high amounts of nitrates. Nitrates are converted into nitric oxide by our bodies. This chemical can lower blood pressure. According to studies, beetroot can moderately control blood pressure; however, more study is necessary. It is still considered to be great for the health of your heart and cardiovascular system.

Another study conducted in 2013 showed the relation between beetroots and improved exercise and performance. According to this study, beetroot can improve activity inactive as well as inactive individuals. But elite athletes showed little to no change.

According to a study conducted in 2010, beetroot juice can enhance the flow of blood in the brain. It is also good for the skin and hair and has many cosmetic benefits.

Beetroot has a distinct color and flavor. It is recommended to consume it raw, but you can also cook it according to the recipe. It is a great addition to salads as it provides taste, color, and crunch. Beetroot juice is another common form in which beetroot can be consumed with ease.

Kale

Kale is considered one of the healthiest leafy vegetables. It contains high amounts of nutrients and is really great for people who are trying to lose weight. Kale contains many medicinal properties as well. Kale is highly versatile, and it can be had in many different forms. It is easy to incorporate in daily meals. It can be eaten raw, fried, or it can be made into soups and salads as well. Thus, kale is one of the best superfoods currently available.

Kale is a member of the cabbage family. Like other cruciferous vegetables, such as broccoli, Brussels sprouts, and cauliflower, kale too is extremely healthy and nutritious. There are many different varieties of kale available in the market. Green and purple varieties are the most popular. The shape of leaves of kale varieties varies a lot. Some have plain leaves, while others have curved and rounded leaves. Curly Kale or Scots Kale is a popular variety of kale that has curly leaves and a stark green color.

Kale is extremely rich in nutrients. A single cup contains high amounts of minerals such as calcium, manganese, potassium, copper, and magnesium. It also contains high amounts of vitamins such as A, K, C, B6. A single cup of kale contains around 6 grams of carbs, 3 grams of proteins, and only 33 calories. Kale contains little to no fat, which makes it great for people who are trying to lose weight. Kale is considered to be one of the most nutrient-dense foods in the world.

Kale is rich in antioxidants like other green leafy vegetables. It contains high amounts of beta-carotene, Quercetin, and Kaempferol. It also contains high amounts of vitamin C, which is good for your immune system. In fact, a cup of kale contains more vitamin C than an orange!

Kale contains high amounts of bile acids, such as sequestrants, which can control your cholesterol level. Thus, kale is really great for the health of your heart and cardiovascular system as well.

Cancer is an extremely terrible disease that can wreak havoc in a person's life. Kale contains many components that can fight cancer efficiently.

Kale contains high amounts of minerals and can thus prevent mineral deficiency. Spinach is another green leafy vegetable that is full of nutrients, but when compared to kale, spinach falls short. Kale is not only rich in minerals, but it is also low in oxalate.

People who are trying to lose weight are often worried about their diet and what to eat and what not to eat. Kale is definitely a great choice for anyone who is trying to lose weight. It is low in calories but can still keep you satiated for a long time.

Spinach

Spinach is a great leafy vegetable that contains high amounts of nutrients. It is dark, leafy, and contains very few calories. It is good for your skin, bones, hair, and heart. It also contains high amounts of iron, protein, minerals, and vitamins. Spinach can help you to control blood sugar levels, improve bone health, and can also lower the risk of cancer significantly. It also contains a variety of minerals that are good for your health.

Spinach has been used by many different cultures since ancient times. It is a staple food of middle-eastern, Mediterranean, and Southeast Asian cultures. It is versatile and can be added to almost any food. It has its own distinct flavor, but it is not overpowering and thus can be mixed with other ingredients with ease. Spinach is also cheap and easy to cook. There are many different ways of cooking spinach, but you can also eat it raw. Spinach is really good for reducing oxidative stress. It is also good for blood pressure levels and optical health as well.

Spinach contains high amounts of insoluble fiber, which is good for weight loss and digestion. It also contains high amounts of lutein, kaempferol, quercetin, nitrates, and zeaxanthin, which are all good for your health.

Spinach contains high amounts of vitamin K1, so people who suffer from kidney stones should avoid it. It is also not recommended for people who are on blood thinners. Other than these people, everyone can consume spinach.

Green Tea

Green tea is a great beverage that contains many different nutrients. It has many health benefits and properties due to the way it is prepared and processed. To make black tea, the tea leaves are fermented, which gives it a distinct taste and color. In the case of green tea, the leaves are steamed. Due to this, the tea leaves do not lose a lot of nutrients and taste. This is why green tea is extremely rich in antioxidants.

Green tea is known to prevent or slow down the growth of cancer. It fights the battle against cancer on all fronts. For instance, it protects the DNA against any damage. It also attacks the cancerous cells. It can even shut down crucial molecules that are responsible for the development of cancer.

According to recent Swedish research, green tea also stops the formation of new blood vessels. These vessels are responsible for spreading tumors.

Green tea can also reduce and repair the damage caused to the liver due to alcohol. It is also good against various diseases, including Parkinson's and rheumatoid arthritis. It also prevents cholesterol from choking blood vessels. Women who drink green tea regularly have better bones than those who don't. Thus, green tea also reduces the risk of osteoporosis in women.

Green tea is full of nutrients, such as antioxidants that are great for the body. These are responsible for enhanced brain function, reduced risk of cancer, and enhanced fat loss as well.

Green tea also contains small amounts of caffeine that can keep you awake for a long time. It also acts as a stimulant and is good for the health of your brain. While the amount of caffeine present in green tea is lower than the amount present in coffee, it is still potent enough to give you efficient results.

Green tea also contains important amino acids, such as L-theanine. This amino acid works in combination with caffeine to improve brain function. Green tea can also boost your metabolism and thus can lead to efficient fat burning. It has other antioxidants that can help you prevent cancer.

There are various bioactive compounds present in green tea, which are good for the health of your brain. They can reduce the effects of Parkinson's and Alzheimer's effectively. These two are the most common neurodegenerative disorders. Green tea contains a high amount of catechins, which can reduce the growth of certain viruses and bacteria. This is turn can reduce infections and can also improve your oral and dental health. It is also effective against halitosis.

In certain controlled trials, it was observed that green tea could also reduce blood sugar levels and thus can reduce the risk of Type 2 diabetes as well. Green tea can also reduce LDL cholesterol. Thus, green tea can help you live longer and look young for a long time as well.

Apples

Apples are one of the best fruits, as they contain no cholesterol or fats. They also contain no sodium and are a great low-calorie snack. Apples are not only delicious, but they are also highly nutritious. Apples contain high amounts of dietary fiber. It is estimated that one medium-sized fruit contains around 5 grams of dietary fiber. Apples are a rich source of soluble fiber, which is good for satiation. This is why apples are often an integral part of the diet of people who are trying to lose weight. Apples keep you feeling full for a long time.

Apples contain high amounts of vitamin C along with fiber. They are also a rich source of polyphenols. Polyphenols have multiple health benefits and are great for your cardiovascular health. Apples also contain nutrients that can help you to lower your cholesterol levels. According to studies, eating apples regularly can also help you lower the risk of Type 2 diabetes.

The type of fiber that is present in apple acts as food for bacteria. These good gut bacteria are essential for digestive health. They are also helpful in the case of heart problems, obesity, and Type 2 diabetes. Apples also contain many different nutrients that can fight cancer efficiently.

Apples also contain high amounts of anti-inflammatory compounds and antioxidants. They can help the regular immune system. These antioxidants are also good for the health of your bones. Apples are also great for your memory as they reduce wear and tear of neurotransmitters.

Flax Seeds

Flax seeds are tiny, but they contain high amounts of nutrients. They are full of omega-3, fiber, fatty acids, antioxidants, lignans, and many different varieties of vitamin B. Only a couple of teaspoons of flax seeds per day can provide you a lot of nutrients and can keep you healthy and fit. Incorporating flax seeds in your daily diet is easy as they can be added to literally any food, including salads, shakes, desserts, etc. Flax seeds and flaxseed oil have both been used for cooking for a long time. A lot of records regarding flax seeds have been found throughout the world.

Flax seeds come from the flowers of the flax plant. They are slightly larger than sesame seeds. They are normally available in shades such as dark brown and golden tan. They are flat and shiny. The seeds have a slightly nutty and earthy flavor, but their flavor often gets overpowered by other flavors when they are used in other dishes.

While flax seeds contain a multitude of nutrients, they are celebrated for being rich in lignans, omega 3, and fiber.

Flax seeds are great for vegetarians and vegans. Normally the best source for omega 3 is salmon, but vegans can get a lot of omega 3 from flaxseed. Flax seeds contain high amounts of ALA, which is a form of omega 3. ALA is good for the health of your heart, and it can also reduce the risk of stroke.

Along with ALA, flax seeds also contain high amounts of lignans. Lignans are a group of ingredients that are highly potent antioxidants. They can help to prevent breast and prostate cancer. They can also slow down the development of other cancers as well.

Flax seeds are great for people who suffer from digestive problems or are trying to lose weight. As flax seeds are full of fiber, they can improve your digestion. A high amount of fiber can also lower cholesterol and can improve the health of your heart as well. Flaxseeds also contain a high amount of insoluble fiber. Insoluble fiber can lower your blood sugar levels significantly — this why doctors often recommend diabetic patients to incorporate flax seeds in their diet.

Flax seeds are also great for people who are trying to lose weight. Flax seeds contain a high amount of fiber, which keeps you full for a long time.

Incorporating flax seeds into your diet is easy. You can either consume raw flax seeds or roasted flax seeds. The easiest way to eat flax seeds is by using them in shakes and salads. You can also consume spoonfuls of flax seeds twice daily. Flaxseed oil/gel is also great for the health of your hair and skin.

Oats

Oats have become really popular in modern times. They are high in nutrients that are available almost everywhere. They are extremely beneficial for our health. Oats are generally 100% whole grains that undergo a very low amount of processing. They contain high amounts of minerals, vitamins, and fiber. They also contain high amounts of beta-glucan. This is a soluble fiber that is good for lower cholesterol reabsorption. Oats also contain low amounts of sodium and a good amount of protein, which makes it great for people trying to lose weight.

According to the FDA review, oats can reduce LDLs, i.e., the lower serum cholesterol levels. This is a result of beta-glucan. This soluble fiber has made oats really popular among masses, especially among people who are trying to lose weight. While oats do help you to lose weight, they are not a 'one-time magic' solution that works instantly. You do need to combine oats with other methods of weight loss.

Oats are low in calories and contain high amounts of proteins and fiber. This makes them great for people trying to lose weight. They contain high amounts of potassium, magnesium, zinc, manganese, copper, thiamine, selenium, and pantothenic acid. They also contain high amounts of phytonutrients such as phytoestrogens, polyphenols, lignins, vitamin R, and protease inhibitors.

According to studies, if individuals who have high cholesterol consume even 3 grams of oat fiber every day (i.e., a bowl of oatmeal), their cholesterol levels can go down by 8-23 percent. Even a 1 percent drop is good for the heart and reduces the risk of developing heart disease. Thus, oats are really good for people who are at risk of developing heart problems.

Oats contain a lot of nutrients that make them exceptionally good for people who are trying to eat healthily and stay fit. They are good for your immune system and can help you tackle a lot of diseases and disorders as well. Oats are available with ease almost everywhere in the world. They are a staple ingredient in many baked goods. Almost all restaurants and breakfast places feature different kinds of oatmeal on their menu.

As said above, there are many different varieties of oats available in the market. Steel-cut oats can bring a lot of texture and flavor to otherwise plain and bland foods.

Oats are extremely versatile, and there are various methods of cooking and eating them. The easiest way to consume oats is in the form of cereals or oatmeal, but you can also consume oats in the form of cookies, cakes, shakes, salads, etc. Oats do not have a strong flavor profile and thus can be mixed with anything.

Hemp Seeds

It may come as a surprise, but it is true, hemp seeds are really good for your health. The scientific name of hemp seeds is Cannabis Sativa. Nowadays, thanks to research, people have realized that hemp seeds are indeed a superfood. They contain high amounts of nutrients that are really good for your body. Many people call hemp seeds to be the most nutritious food available for consumption. Hemp seeds are great for weight loss as they contain a high amount of fiber. They can help you stay full for a long time. They can also reduce your hunger pangs and thus ultimately control your weight. Eating hemp seeds is easy; just add a couple of teaspoons to your morning meal. Eating hemp seeds in the morning will help you stay satiated for a long time throughout the day.

Hemp seeds can be eaten raw, whole, toasted, or roasted. Nowadays, they are also available in various flavors to make them more palatable. You can use these seeds in various ways. You can also use the oil prepared from these seeds. The leftover stuff remaining after extracting oil from hemp seeds is quite nutrient-rich as well. Hemp is as healthy as any green vegetable. The health benefits of hemp and hemp seeds have now been proven by science as well.

Hemp seeds can efficiently reduce the risk of heart disease. Heart diseases and disorders are the two leading causes of death all around the world. According to research, hemp seeds can reduce the risk of developing heart diseases and disorders. Hemp seeds contain high amounts of amino acids. These acids produce nitric oxide in the body. This nitric oxide is good for the health of your blood vessels as it relaxes them and thus lowers and regulates your blood pressure. This, in turn, reduces the risk of heart disorders.

Omega 6, omega 3, and amino acids are essential for a healthy immune system. Hemp seeds are rich sources of these three nutrients and are thus great for your immune system. Amino acids are also good for the health of your skin. Hemp seed oil can work wonders for all your skin problems, including signs of aging, dark spots, acne, etc.

Hemp seeds are a boon for women suffering from menopause and PMS. It can effectively tackle the symptoms of PMS. According to studies, the hormone prolactin causes the symptoms associated with PMS. Hemp seeds contain a high amount of gamma linoleum acid, which can tackle prolactin by producing prostaglandin el.

Hemp seeds also contain a high amount of fiber. They contain both insoluble and soluble fiber in an 80:20 ratio. This makes hemp seeds really good for your digestive health.

Hemp seeds do not contain any trans fats, which makes them great for people who are trying to lose weight. Thus, including hemp seeds in your regular diet will help you become fit, healthy, and young. If you do not like the taste of hemp seeds, try using the flavored ones.

Goji Berries

Goji berries have become one of the most celebrated superfoods now. They are reddish-orange berries that grow on the wolfberry plant. These plants are native to China. They are kind of tart but also have an inherent sweetness. Goji berries are more popular for their health benefits. They contain high amounts of antioxidants and a variety of nutrients as well.

Ancient Chinese medicine schools have been using goji berries for thousands of years for a variety of ailments and problems. Recently, goji berries and their immense health benefits have been introduced to the western world, which is why they have become a staple in health food stores.

Goji berries contain a high amount of vitamin C, even more than oranges. It also contains a high amount of selenium, calcium, iron, potassium, and zinc.

Goji berries also contain a high number of carotenoids, such as beta-carotene. It is good for the health of your eyes and optical nerves. It also contains a high amount of fiber, which is good for your digestive system. Goji berries can reduce fatigue and stress by giving your energy boosts. They contain a high amount of melatonin, which makes them great for people who suffer from insomnia or other sleep-related problems.

Goji berries are also rich in protein. They contain around 12-14% protein. They are the right combination of taste and health. In the west, these berries are generally available in dried form. High quality dried berries are soft and fleshy.

Goji berries are versatile, and there are many different ways you can use them. Some people prefer to eat them right out of the bag. They can also be mixed with other dried fruits, seeds, and nuts. You can also add them to smoothies and shakes. Some people also like to toss some berries in their salads. This makes the salad look and taste good.

Coconut

Coconut is a great superfood that can help you become fit and healthy. It is a versatile fruit that can be used in a variety of forms. Some of the most common forms include dried coconut, raw coconut meat, coconut oil, coconut water, coconut milk, etc. Coconuts have been grown and used since ancient times in various tropical regions around the world. Now they are gaining rapid popularity all over the world thanks to their immense culinary versatility and numerous health benefits.

While other fruits are full of carbs, coconut contains high amounts of fats. They are also a rich source of protein, vitamins, and minerals. Coconut contains a high amount of manganese, which is good for the health of your bones. It also metabolizes proteins, cholesterol, and carbs efficiently.

Coconuts are also rich in iron and copper. They also contain selenium. Selenium is an essential antioxidant that keeps your cells healthy.

Coconut contains high amounts of MCT or medium-chain triglycerides. Our body uses these fats for instant energy and does not store them. Thus, coconut is good for people who are trying to lose weight.

Coconut is also great for the health of your heart. It was found that people who live on Polynesian islands rarely get heart diseases and disorders. This is because their diet is rich in coconuts. According to certain studies, if you consume coconut oil, it may help you to reduce belly fat. This is especially great for people who are trying to lose weight. According to studies, coconut oil can also reduce cholesterol levels.

Coconut contains high amounts of fiber and fat but a low amount of carbs. This combination is great for your blood sugar levels. It can reduce your blood sugar levels efficiently.

Coconuts contain arginine. Arginine is an essential amino acid that improves pancreatic activity. It plays an important role in the regulation of blood sugar levels. Eating coconut also affects the beta cells present in the pancreas, which are responsible for the production of insulin.

Due to the high fiber content of coconut meat, you can also lose weight and stay satiated for a long time.

Coconuts are full of various antioxidants. Most of these antioxidants are phenolic compounds such as caffeic acid, gallic acid, salicylic acid, p-coumaric acid, etc. All these acids are good for the health of your body as they tackle free radicals.

It also contains a high number of polyphenols, which reduces the oxidation of LDL. Oxidized LDL leads to the formation of plaque in arteries.

Coconuts are extremely versatile, and they can be eaten in a variety of ways. Shaved or flaked coconuts are great for savory dishes. Shaved coconut is a great addition to rice, stews, soups, curries, etc. Certain brands of shaved coconut contain sugar, so it is best to avoid them if you want to lose weight.

Shredded coconut is great for desserts and baked goods. Raw coconut can add a really brilliant tropical flavor to any dish. If you are allergic to gluten, then you can replace wheat flour with coconut flour. This flower is also suitable for Paleo diet followers.

Coconut oil can be used for cooking, frying, baking, and roasting as well.

Garlic

Garlic has been used for its taste enhancing and medicinal properties since ancient times. Hippocrates, the father of modern medicine, used to prescribe garlic for a variety of ailments. Now modern science has confirmed and proved its health benefits.

Garlic is a member of the onion or Allium family. The members of this family, such as onions, shallots, etc. contain a lot of sulfur compounds that are responsible for the health benefits. One such compound is allicin. Along with allicin, other compounds that make garlic healthy include diallyl disulfide and s-allyl cysteine. Garlic is great for weight loss as it contains a very low number of calories. One clove of raw garlic has:

- 2% of daily manganese
- 2% of daily vitamin B6
- 1% of daily vitamin C
- 1% of daily selenium
- 0.06 grams of fiber

It also contains moderate amounts of copper, calcium, potassium, iron, phosphorus, and vitamin B1.

It contains only 4.5 calories and 1 gram of carbs. It also contains around 0.2 grams of protein. Garlic is good for the health of your immune system. It is effective against the common cold as well. It is also used to treat cough and sore throat.

Garlic is supposed to be great for the health of your heart as well. It is good for hypertension and high blood pressure, as well. Garlic can also reduce the levels of cholesterol and thus reduce the risk of heart diseases. It is really effective against LDL cholesterol.

Garlic is rich in antioxidants. These antioxidants can tackle free radicals and prevent oxidative damage as well. These antioxidants can also improve your immune system. According to some sources, garlic can also target Alzheimer's and dementia as well.

Garlic can also increase your longevity. It can tackle many different infections, as well as chronic diseases. Garlic also has detoxifying effects that can prevent organ damage by getting rid of harmful chemicals from the body. Another thing that makes garlic really great for health is that it can make your bones strong. It reduces bone damage, especially in the case of women. It can reduce the occurrence of osteoporosis in women.

Garlic is a versatile food item that can be incorporated into various recipes. It goes great with bread, soups, and sauces. Garlic has a strong taste, and thus, it can make otherwise bland food taste good. Garlic can be used in a variety of forms. The most commonly used forms are cloves. It is also possible to use garlic in the form of pastes and powders. Nowadays, garlic oil is used in a lot of cuisines as well.

Garlic can cause halitosis if used improperly. It is recommended to avoid using garlic if you are allergic to it. Garlic is also not recommended for people who are on blood-thinners.

Nicholas Bjorn

Chapter 5 – 8 Reasons Why You Are Not Losing Body Fat

Collectively, we spend years of our lives trying to shed those extra pounds of body fat but have little to no success. We go on diet after diet, our weight yo-yoing up and down and we ride on a rollercoaster that has way too much roll in it. We try to shed the fat when we are motivated but still fall apart when we see a plate of fresh warm cookies. Unfortunately, this is why so many New Year's resolutions wind up discarded and gym memberships get ignored. While we might have a common goal in mind, losing fat, it is not an easy thing to achieve satisfactorily.

If you have been playing the same game and haven't yet succeeded, you are more than likely making a couple of mistakes. Below I am going to talk about the 8 most common mistakes that people make when they are trying to lose fat:

Mistake Number 1 – You are eating too much

This might seem like an obvious on but so many people seriously do not know how many calories they are eating. A salad might seem like a low calorie option but you may actually be munching your way through 600 calories. Salad dressings, sauces, ketchups and oils are all loaded with calories that you don't always see or think about, especially if you are not a regular cook at home.

We are always told to eat less calories than we are burning but this simplifies matters too much. This would work if you, for example, ate 1500 calories worth of cheesecake every day and burned 2000 calories. But, the one thing the human body can't do is be a calculator. What matters is not how many calories but the type of calories you are eating. If you eat a diet that is made up of carbohydrates only, you won't burn any fat, whereas if you eat less of the carbs and more protein, fat and the right carbs, you are on to a winning combination for burning fat and building up muscle.

Most people find that a ratio of 40% carbs, 40% protein and 20% fat works perfectly to burn off that fat. However, that may not work for all so you will need to do your research and work out what is best for you. Some people have to reduce their carb limit even lower to be successful but, if you have to do that, boost up your good fat intake to allow your body an alternative source of energy to burn.

Mistake Number 2 – You are not eating enough protein

Protein isn't just for building and repairing your muscle tissue. Recent studies have showed that, on two groups of women who were overweight, both of whom consumed the same number of calories per day, the group that consumed 128 g protein every day lost more weight than the group who consumed just 68 g protein per day.

Protein makes you feel fuller for much longer and stops you from grazing throughout the day and from eating too much at your main meals. A high protein diet can also affect the glucose levels, blood lipids and muscle to fat ratio in the body in a positive manner. Protein is an excellent fat loss macro but you will not see instant results by adding protein shakes to your diet. Fat burning is not instant; it takes dedication and consistently following the meal plan to make a difference. What you can do is add high protein foods to your meals and cut down on the bad carbs foods – you will see the results in time.

Mistake Number 3 – You are drinking too much

You really only need to drink water. You can have tea or coffees, occasionally milk but stop the stream of sugar-filled drinks. All they are doing is undoing the good work the rest of your food is doing. One pumpkin spice latte can contain over 300 calories, and that is just in one drink! That is not doing your body any good at all – all you are doing is making your fat loss goas harder to attain.

Alcohol is also a bad call. While a beer or a glass of wine every now and again isn't going to make much difference, you must stop the binging at weekends. Alcohol is high in calories, these are stored by your body as fat, and it also causes an impairment to your judgment. Instead of eating a good healthy choice, the booze will tell you that a big pate of cheesy chips is just the right thing to eat.

Mistake Number 4 – You think that healthy foods have no calories

Everything has calories in it, regardless of how healthy it is. If you eat too much, you will struggle to shed the fat. Of course, you need to eat whole foods but eating too much organic peanut butter is still overeating whichever you look at it. Two examples of healthy foods that are significantly high in calories are seeds and nuts. They contain micronutrients, omega 3 and phytogens that are absolutely wonderful for your health but are excessively high in calories. Don't avoid them; just stick to eating a small handful at a time.

Mistake Number 5 – Your training regime is not intensive enough

While it is important for complete beginners to start off slowly, you should gradually up your game, as you become more and more used to the gym machines, weights and the actual exercise itself. Start to push yourself harder and harder – if you get comfortable doing your training, your weight loss will simply plateau. If you are not breaking a sweat through your exercise, you are not working out hard enough. If you are not sweating, you are not burning fat and your heart rate is not working to your benefit.

If you are looking to burn fat, you need to create an extreme energy demand so that your body is able to change. Lifting the same old weights time and time again will not help you to burn fat and you won't be gaining any real benefits from your physical activity.

Mistake Number 6 – You are doing too much low intensity cardio training

Ok, so I just told you to up the intensity of your workout and now I'm telling you off for doing too much of something that isn't intensive. Cardio is not a form of resistance training. It is a completely different type of fitness and a two-hour slog on the treadmill is not going to give you the results that an hour of heavy lifting will.

If you want your cardio to work, do full body workouts that include a short rest period. By using your whole body and taking shorter breaks, your cardiovascular system and your muscular system are being challenged.

Mistake Number 7 – You are stressed out

Stress is one of the biggest and most silent killers. Stress causes your body to produce cortisol in levels way beyond what is normal. This can be responsible to an increase in fat storage in the body and many other negative consequences. Even if your diet and your training regime are spot-on, if you re stressed, you will not achieve your goals.

The key is to relax and, although that is easier said than done, if you can learn some deep breathing, meditation, or yoga and incorporate it every day in your diet, you will see a significant change in your overall health and in your physique

Mistake 8 – You are not sleeping enough

Sleek deprivation also raises cortisol levels and, when you are lacking in sleep; your insulin sensitivity is also reduced. Together, these two problems are not good news for anyone who wants to burn fat. Sleep is a priority in your life. You cannot possibly party all night and expect to function well the next day. Aim for 8 hours of good sleep every single night. Don't drink alcohol, don't use your tablet, mobile phone or watch TV for at least an hour before you go to bed, eliminate caffeine in the evenings and give yourself time to relax in the evenings.

Nicholas Bjorn

Chapter 6 – Eat Right For Weight Loss

From what most of you have read in numerous articles and papers and, of course, the grand old Internet, there are about a gazillion diets to follow. People religiously begin one in the month of January and drop out mid-way due to sheer fatigue, exhaustion, and the primal urge to eat. Almost all diets work in the short term - by eliminating one or more crucial food groups, such as carbs or fat or vegetables or any combination of the groups. That is why, by forcing yourself to eat fewer calories per meal, you definitely lose weight in the beginning. But later on, as your body demands the lost nutrition, you begin bingeing on unhealthy foods and snacks and promptly gain all the weight you managed to lose. That's sad, really. But there's no denying it - you can't fool your body.

But there's a way out. You really don't have to starve or deprive yourself of eating your favorite foods. You can do that and STILL beat the escalating calories. Is it magic? Is it like entering the world of wizards? Is it some alternate realm of reality?

Not really. It's a basic, most fundamental fact of biology. Losing weight happens simply because you consume fewer calories than you burn. That's it. No complicated charts and figures. If you eat less and expend more calories, you lose weight. How this happens is important.

First, we need to understand what a calorie is and what all the fuss is about it.

Simply put, a calorie is a unit of energy. All our foods and drinks give us some kind of energy, the fuel for our body. Carbohydrates, fats, proteins, minerals, and vitamins - all have calories. How much energy they give out is measured by calories. Each day, our body requires a certain number of calories for its normal function - for your heartbeats, brain activity, body functions, etc. So, just in order to EXIST, you expend calories. This is called the Total Daily Energy Expenditure or TDEE. For example, if you are a 40-year-old female, weighing 140 pounds and standing 5"5' tall, you burn 1350 calories by just existing. Similarly, the calorie expenditure of a 30-year-old male, weighing 240 pounds and being 6 feet tall is around 2300. Get a general idea?

Basal Metabolic Rate (BMR)

BMR is basically the number of calories required by your body for its daily function. This base number of calories is required for involuntary functions of the body, such as breathing, pumping of the heart, digestion, etc. According to the Academy of Nutrition and Dietetics, your BMR should not drop below 1200. If it does, it starts affecting your metabolism in a bad way. Muscle mass begins to decrease; body fat falls below acceptable levels, circulation and pulse rate is affected, brain function is affected. Your overall health declines, which is precisely what you DO NOT want.

Factors such as gender, weight, and height affect this number. For a rough estimate, about two-thirds of the calories you eat go into the daily function of your body. The other third portion goes into the motion-related activities of your body. This also depends on the activity levels of your body.

Sedentary Lifestyle: BMR x 1.2

Slightly Active: BMR x 1.375

Moderately Active: BMR x 1.55

Very Active: BMR x 1.725

Now, let us show you an example. You are a 35-year-old male, weighing 200 pounds and standing 72 inches tall (six feet).

Let's use some numbers:

Suppose you're male, 35 years old, weigh 200 pounds and are six feet even (72 inches).

BMR= 1882 calories

If you are a sedentary person, this number jumps to 2258. That means you need that many calories just to sustain yourself on a daily basis, do your tasks, work, etc. If you are a moderately active person, your TDEE comes to 2917.

Now see the difference between being sedentary and moderately active. It amounts to 659 calories. That equals one whole meal! And that is why I wrote in the beginning- we tend to underestimate how much we are eating, but overestimate how much we are expending.

When you eat something, your body has three categories to decide where all those calories will go:

- for fuel-burning
- for rebuilding muscles
- for storing as fat

When you expend as many calories as you consume, you reach something called a "calorie equilibrium." No more, no less. Just a pleasant state of homeostasis. If you want to lose weight, you will need to eat fewer calories. This forces your body to hit the calorie reserve it has to burn fuel.

Now, when you eat more and burn fewer calories, the body does not need the extra calories it just ate. So, they are stored as fat, a.k.a, weight gain. And when you begin to see sense and burn off those extra calories or eat a calorie deficit, you lose weight. Simple?

Sure, in theory. But life isn't this simple, right. We are super amazing at underplaying the amount of food we eat and overestimating the rate at which we burn it off. Human nature, really! The so-called cheat days between exercise regimes, the accidental over-eating of your favorite dessert at a party, or someone's birthday - these are just some of the umpteen excuses we give ourselves when confronted with the reality.

Metabolism and Weight Loss

Your resting metabolism slows down when you lose weight. This is a simple concept. Because there is less of you to fuel and process, your metabolism doesn't have to work that hard to keep your bodily functions intact and functioning properly. When you lose weight, you also lose some water, lean tissue, and fat. If you weigh less, it will have less weight to carry around; the heart will have to pump less, etc. The body will, therefore, burn fewer calories than it did when you carried all that extra weight.

If you look at estimates from a calorie calculator, here's how much the resting calorie burn is for three different weights.

- 2600 calories for 300 lbs
- 2300 calories for 250 lbs
- 2000 calories for 200 lbs.

See the difference? By weighing just 50 pounds less, you strike off 300 calories from your metabolism. But here's where things get interesting. There is something called "adaptive thermogenesis." It basically means that the body keeps adjusting itself to the number of calories consumed and burnt per day, and the process it takes to preserve the body fat within.

Our body is constantly wondering if it will get the next meal or not. Because it does that, it has a tendency to store the calories as surplus - just in case the Earth is invaded, and we are left without supplies. That is why even though people seem to lose a few pounds, they have to make a consistent and lifelong effort to keep the extra kilos off. Many other factors - such as environmental changes, psychological elements, medication, depression, emotional pain, anxiety, and other issues can trigger or change eating patterns.

Now, instead of worrying about calories every single time you look at food, it's far, far better to eat the healthy and right kind of foods in the first place. For example - protein (meat, legumes), carbohydrates (brown or white rice, quinoa, wheat), fruit and vegetables, nuts, dairy (if you are not lactose intolerant). Just keep eating these foods and stay happy, full, and healthy for a long, long time. These wholesome foods keep us full for a much longer time, yet aren't that calorie-dense. If you do this over a consistent period of time, you will lose weight.

So, what can you eat to lose weight in a healthy manner?

Protein

As you have learned already, protein is the building block for our skin, hair, and muscles. If eaten properly, it makes for a very filling and delicious food group. Generally speaking, you should eat about 1 gram of protein per lb. of bodyweight. Guzzling a can of energy drink will fill you up for about ten minutes. And leave you with loads of unwanted calories. The same amount of calories can be obtained from a good serving of chicken. Healthier, right? Because protein requires energy to metabolize, a high protein diet can be key for a calorie deficit. It fights the primary cause of weight gain - cravings. Protein can be found in meat, legumes, fowl, eggs, fish, etc. But try to keep the upper limit at 250 grams, because too much of anything can also cause problems.

Vegetables

No, pizza is not a vegetable. Real vegetables are rich in nutrients and calorie-light. That means you can eat a lot of these and feel full but are very unlikely to gain weight. Every meal should have at least two servings of differently colored vegetables - the more color, the better. Seasonal vegetables work best. Broccoli, spinach, cauliflower, radish, Brussels sprouts, kale, zucchini, cucumber, carrots, onions, potatoes, asparagus, etc. are some veggies to get you interested!

Fat

Yes, I said fat. Fat has always been vilified, but healthy fats work wonders for your body and especially for your skin. Foods such as avocado, nuts, olive oil, peanut butter, whole milk, grass-fed butter, etc. contain healthy fat needed by the body. Consume these in small amounts to reap maximum benefits and also lose weight in the process.

The Grain is a Go-Go

Instead of highly processed junk food like pizza, burgers, patties, ready to eat meals and soups, cakes and cookies, go for whole grains. Choose whole-wheat pasta, brown bread, bran, rye crackers, etc. These will fill you up and keep you satiated for a longer time.

Minimize Processed Food

If it's not growing on a tree or swimming in the sea or pulled up from the Earth, don't bother eating it. Processed food is designed to be super tasty but, in reality, contains a whole lot of preservatives and additives. It does make people addicted to it.

Oversee Liquid Calories

Fruit juices and those who say "enriched fruit or energy water" are nothing but sugar in a liquid form. All of your sodas and colas also fall into this category. Liquid calories account for why people can't seem to lose weight even after switching to healthier diets. Even seemingly harmless coffee orders contain lots of cream and sugar. These drinks and beverages have no fiber and only sugar inside them, which wreaks havoc with our bodily systems. Alcohol also does the same - provide empty calories and a hangover which nobody wants. Sugar not only causes obesity but a host of other diseases. If you want your weight loss to work, drink lots of water, black or green tea, or sparkling water. That's it, no sugary beverages.

Drink More Water

This is such an important point; it has been dealt with in another chapter in the book. Drinking water has been found to increase the number of calories you burn. Studies have shown that drinking about eight glasses of water per day is equal to having burnt about 96 extra calories. Sweet deal! Of course, WHEN you drink, it is also important. Drinking water half an hour before meals help reduce hunger, and thus, you eat less, creating a calorie deficit. Also, drinking water half an hour after meals are also beneficial to digestion.

Because the thirst and hunger centers are located so close to each other in the hypothalamus, most of the time, in between meals, we tend to feel hungry when, in fact, we are THIRSTY. Drinking water will curb this pang of false hunger, and you will eat properly when the actual mealtime comes around.

Condiments and Accompaniments

If your healthy broccoli, pear and carrot salad has a generous overdose of ketchup and mayo over it, or if you dunk everything in heavy sauces and dips, the actual nutritional value becomes less. Keep an eye on what you put on your veggies and meats.

Smaller Meals

Food nutrition experts also recommend that you eat smaller meals and pace them throughout the day. This keeps your blood sugar levels in check and also stops you from overindulging on unhealthy snacks.

Smart Substitutions

Don't want to eat salad by itself? Add some vinegar, soy sauce, and basil for an instant livening up of the situation. Homemade salsa and hummus, mustard paste, homemade white butter for your jacket potatoes, basil and cilantro, lemon, and vinegar are all healthy complements and dressings for your pasta, salad, and toppings.

What Else Can I Do?

Predetermine your Meals

I know it sounds like a boring and tedious activity. But picture this - you're home tired after a long day's work, and maybe managed to squeeze in some exercise in between. But you're too tired to cook, so you just order some pizza and a soda, and all your hard work go down the drain. Pre-plan and pre-cook your meals and bung them in the freezer. It makes a world of difference in your weight loss journey.

Strength Train

I can't stress this enough. When you lift weights, you force your muscles to break down. And when you rest and eat properly, the muscles rebuild themselves and take the fuel from the stores available in your body. That means, even as you are resting, you are burning calories. It's a win-win all the way - as you keep getting stronger, your muscles become bigger, and you keep losing body fat. This is also an important aspect of losing weight and maintaining it and is discussed in a separate chapter.

Calorie Deficit

Consistently maintain a calorie deficit. You can also mix and match your exercise routines to include cardio, strength training, Zumba, Pilates, yoga, etc. and continue with your healthy weight loss journey.

Step Up!

Even if you can't find the time to strength train, you can always start walking. That remains the best and most natural exercise ever designed for the body. Move constantly. Park your car a few hundred yards from your office or home. Take the stairs at work. Walk back from the supermarket. Run around with your dog or your neighbor's dog. March in place while watching advertisements. Just keep moving it.

Close your Kitchen at Night

Late-night snacking in front of the TV, eating because you don't have anything else to do or simply dipping your hand inside the cookie jar every time you enter the kitchen - these are just some of the ways in which you pile on unnecessary pounds. Set a time for your meals and stick to it. Get into the habit of closing up the kitchen after a set time, say 9 p.m. No going into the kitchen or fridge after that. If it helps, brush your teeth an hour after eating. The minty taste will let you forget any mindless snacking you might want to indulge in.

Controlling your Immediate Environment

If your fridge is always stocked with pastries, cakes, sodas, pizzas, and the like, it's very unlikely that you will reach for a bag of cauliflower or carrots when there is an appetizing cheese burst pizza staring at you. Make it a point to stock your pantry and fridge with healthy foods - vegetables, fruit, healthy cuts of meat, nuts, olive oil, whole grains, popcorn, lemon water, etc. so that when you feel the urge to snack or make yourself a meal, you reach out for real food.

One Step at a Time

I get it. You're ambitious and want to lose ten pounds by this Saturday. But if you cut back on your favorite foods, begin a vigorous strength training regime, say bye-bye to alcohol and keep moving all the time - you will most definitely hit a plateau very soon. Take it slowly. Cut back on one unhealthy snack per week. Or have one glass of wine in two weeks. Go for a walk first instead of lifting weights straight away. Take it slowly and steadily.

Check Food Labels

Whenever buying something from the market, be sure to check the nutrition label on the back. If it lists more than ten chemicals and just one or two real food names, chuck it back on the shelf. It's not worth eating it. For example - potato chips should be just that; Potatoes, oil, and salt rather than some twenty triglycerides and ten preservatives shown on the label.

Forgive Yourself

If you ate unhealthy food at one meal, it's okay. It's not the end of the world. Get back on track with your next meal.

You can use some popular apps to keep track of how many calories you are consuming. My Fitness Pal, Fat Secret, and Lose It are three of the most popular ones right now.

Of course, you can't be tracking your food for the rest of your life. But, when you're starting out, it helps to know how much you are eating. That will help you see if you are going overboard with some food groups or ignoring something else completely. Portion sizes also matter here. Let's show you an example.

One pound of fat is equal to something like 3500 calories. So, if you wish to lose one pound of fat per week, you need to eat 500 calories less per day. You can do that either by cutting out 500 calories or burning them through exercise. And arguably, it is much more difficult to increase time for activity levels than it is to reduce calorie consumption. Let's face it - if given a choice, which would you pick? Incorporating thirty minutes or more of exercise time in your schedule or giving up and substituting a food group in your diet?

You guessed it.

Let's take 200 calories as a measure. 200 calories of broccoli would fill up a dinner plate. The same 200 calories are found in half a Snickers bar. How many people you know would prefer eating broccoli to a bar of chocolate? And is it easier to eat a full plate of broccoli than a tempting half bar of yummy chocolate? And who the heck ever eats HALF a bar of chocolate?

That is why you need to eat REAL foods.

Nicholas Bjorn

Chapter 7 – Planning Your Meals

Meal planning may seem to be quite a difficult task, but it really isn't. It is easy and doable if you know and understands what you are doing. In simple terms, meal planning means planning your meals for the week and keeping things ready for these meals. This way, you can save a lot of time and money. Meal planning can be divided into three sections:

- Select the recipes
- Shop for the ingredients
- Prepare the ingredients

Many people find meal planning difficult because many myths that are prevalent about it. For instance, a lot of people believe that you need to plan meals by noting them down in huge binders, which you need to lug around all the time. But this is false; you can make simple meals in Google Docs or any notepad application on your phone. If you do not like using your phone for lists, you can also make simple lists on paper and post it on your fridge.

Many people also think that meal planning is only suitable for large families. But this is false. You can make meal plans for yourself as well. This is especially recommended if you are trying to lose weight or are an extremely busy person. It is also recommended for people who are trying to save money.

Meal planning does not take a lot of work, especially if you have the basics ready. Once you have the basics ready, you can make meal plans for every week in less than an hour.

Meal plans are extremely flexible, and you can change and experiment according to your needs and desires. Nothing is set in stone in the world of meal plans.

Beginning a Meal Plan

Before making a plan, you need to ask yourself:

Why do I need a meal plan?

There are no wrong answers to the above question, but focusing on the reason will allow you to concentrate effectively. In the beginning, keep your reasons and meal plans simple. You can increase the difficulty level with time and experience.

Once you have understood your reason behind meal planning, you can now start with the plan itself. As said above, the first step for meal planning is choosing recipes.

Choosing Recipes

Choosing recipes is a simple task if you know the reason behind your meal plan. For instance, if you are making meal plans because you want to lose weight, it is recommended to choose only healthy recipes. Similarly, if you are making meal plans because you are trying to cut down your expenses, then you should choose recipes that do not require a lot of exotic or expensive ingredients. Thus, you need to focus on the reason behind your meal plan all the time. Never choose recipes randomly. Similarly, avoid making meal plans a day before (at least in the beginning.) Give yourself at least three days to make a meal plan and prepare for it.

If you eat out frequently, add these outings to your meal plan. Once you decide the days and meals, you can move on to the recipes. It is recommended to choose recipes according to your schedule. For instance, if you are generally the busiest on Thursdays, you can either opt for a simple recipe, or you can opt for a recipe that can be made in a slow cooker. This way, you can just add the ingredients to the cooker in the morning and let it cook over low temperature until you return. If you work late on Mondays, you can make more food on Sunday and carry it the next day.

Once you have noted down the recipes, it is now time to get the ingredients.

Ingredients

To make the shopping easy, it is recommended to make two-ingredient lists- a master list and a grocery list. Two lists may sound to be a lot more work than one single list, but making a master list will help you a lot in the long term. The master list will help you keep a stock of fresh and dried ingredients in your pantry, and you won't have to buy them every week.

Master List

In this, add the ingredients that are used in almost all the recipes. You can also add ingredients that are generally purchased in bulk on this list. Try to avoid easily perishable ingredients to this list.

Grocery List

In this list, add anything that can be stored for at least a couple of days. This should include vegetables, dairy, eggs, etc.

Once you have collected the ingredients, the next step in meal planning is preparing them.

Keeping your ingredients prepared is a great way to save time and money. Keeping things prepared is especially great for people who want to avoid working on weekends. Keeping things prepared can help you avoid frustration and fatigue. It will allow you to have more free time for yourself. It is recommended to set aside a few hours on Sunday (or any other day that you are free) and prepare your ingredients according to your meal plan. For instance, if you plan to make salads on Monday or Tuesday, it is recommended to chop some things and refrigerate them. Similarly, if you plan to make pasta or any similar product, you can keep the ingredients for the sauce, such as garlic, etc. ready. Keeping things clean can also save you a lot of time.

Meal plans are simple and effective if you know how to craft them and follow them successfully.

Chapter 8 – The Importance of Water

Water, water everywhere; all the boards did shrink,

Water, water everywhere, nor any drop to drink

The Rime of the Ancient Mariner

Water is everywhere around us, isn't it? That gorgeous pool, those tantalizing lakes and ponds, those mighty seas and majestic oceans of the planet. Over 80 percent of the planet is basically water. And it's the same case with our bodies too. Water makes up a whopping 65 to 70 percent of our bodies. Two atoms of hydrogen, one of oxygen. And it powers the planet. It's not only vital for life to survive and thrive. Going without it for as little as three days will send you into an irreversible spiral of decline.

Now, why is this compound so essential to our health?

Water performs some of the most important functions of the human body: flushing out waste products, regulating body temperature, keeping homeostasis going on properly, aiding brain functions, and more.

Benefits of Drinking Water

Creation of Saliva

Do you know how dry and irritable the mouth gets when you have a fever or some other disease that dries up your mouth? You miss your saliva terribly during those times. Saliva is nothing but water, mucus, and enzymes that break down your food and keep your mouth healthy and germ-free. If you drink water regularly, your body produces enough saliva for proper function. A dry mouth usually indicates dehydration.

Regulation of Body Temperature

Every time you breathe or blink, you lose water through the pores of your skin and eyes. Hydration of the body is vital for the proper regulation of your body temperature. You lose more water through sweat when you exercise or live in hot environments. Sweating keeps your body cool, but the temperature will rise if the loss of water is not replenished. So, keep drinking water to keep your basal metabolic temperature right.

Protection of Tissues, Joints, and Spinal Cord

Water acts as a lubricant and cushions your bones and joints from everyday jarring and bumping around. It eases their function.

Waste Removal

Water is like a carrier of waste material outside your body. By way of sweating, urination, and defecation, water helps flush out toxic waste from your body. Not doing so will result in painful constipation, kidney problems, kidney stones, metabolic breakdown, and a slow build-up of toxins in the body. A build-up of waste in the body can result in bloating and gas in the stomach. People may also feel very lethargic. Generous doses of water throughout the day can help curb this problem.

Maximize Physical Activities and Exertions

During physical activity, a lot of water is lost due to perspiration. Athletes may lose up to 6 to 10 percent of body weight during rigorous training. Drinking plenty of water during such activities helps keep the body cool and energized. Not being hydrated affects your strength and stamina for sports and physical activity. If you exercise in the heat, without drinking adequate water, you may be in danger of serious medical maladies such as heat stroke, hyperthermia, low blood pressure, etc.

Prevention of Constipation

Fiber is a must to have smooth and easy bowel movements. But water aids immensely in the process too. If you don't drink water throughout the day, you might have constipation. The only way out is to drink a couple of glasses of water, wait for an hour or so and then go to the restroom. You will find that the bowel movement is now significantly easier.

Aids in Digestion

Drinking water half an hour before and after meals has been proven to have a positive effect on weight loss and digestion. When you have it before eating, you feel less hungry and eat less. When you drink water half an hour after meals, it won't interfere with the natural digestive processes and helps churn the food easily.

Nutrient Absorption

Water also helps your body to absorb nutrients, vitamins, minerals from food, and delivers these important components to the rest of the body for its building and strengthening activities.

Weight Loss

There are numerous studies linking weight loss and water consumption. While dieting or exercising or just eating healthy, drinking water in adequate amounts also amounts to losing extra pounds.

Fights off Illnesses

Drinking enough water is a natural remedy to ward off diseases like kidney stones, urinary tract infections, hypertension, etc. Water is also a carrier of essential nutrients and vitamins throughout the body, so whatever you eat will be distributed well.

Boosts Energy

Metabolism is also affected by water or lack of it. Drinking water activates the metabolic levels, which, in turn, boosts the energy levels. Studies have shown that as little as 500 ml. of water can increase the metabolism by about 30 percent.

Mood Enhancer

I'm sure you've had bad days, or know of people who became grumpy for no reason at all. Dehydration is also a cause of these kinds of mood swings. It results in fatigue, anxiety, and grumpiness. A bit of water will do the trick!

Skin Lover

We all know the benefits of water for our skin. As the water flushes out toxins from the body, the water which goes into our cells plumps them up. This, in turn, plumps up the skin cells and surfaces and also promotes collagen production, resulting in fewer wrinkles and a more youthful you!

Prevention of Overall Dehydration

We all know how dangerous dehydration is. Severe dehydration can result in kidney failure, brain swelling, seizure, and other body dysfunction. Water helps prevent all these situations. Keep drinking enough water at intervals to sustain a healthy body.

How Much Water Should I Drink?

According to the National Academies of Sciences, Engineering, and Medicine, these are the guidelines for water intake for most people:

Around 125 ounces each day for men and 93 ounces for women. Of course, it all varies depending on the type of work one does and the environment one lives in. Food gives us about 20 percent of our daily intake of water. Everything else depends on how much water and how many water-based drinks you ingest throughout the day.

The color of your urine and thirst you experience are also indicators of your hydration levels. Pale yellow-colored urine is a good indication, while dark yellow means you need to drink more water.

Keep a bottle of water with you and drink from it at regular intervals. As a rule of thumb, aim to drink at least three to four liters of water in a day. Of course, if you end up drinking too much water, that will cause irreparable damage to your body and brain. Just drink enough to sustain and maintain good metabolism.

Water and its Many Forms

Water is just that, right? Plain old boring water? But what about juices, sodas, smoothies, colas, sugary teas, etc.? Sure, they are hydrating and feel particularly great on a hot day, but they also contain enormous quantities of sugar and unwanted calories. Coffee and tea are diuretics - they make you lose water. Alcohol also gives the impression of being hydrating, but it actually has the opposite effect. The same goes for sports drinks. Though they contain electrolytes and other energy-giving substances, they also contain sugar and salt, which is more than the recommended amount. Pay attention to the number of such drinks when you do consume them.

The Role of Water in Weight Loss

Many studies have highlighted the correlation between drinking water and weight loss. Let us see how it does that:

Burns More Calories

When you drink more water, it increases the number of calories burnt by the body, also known as the "resting energy expenditure" of the body. Some studies have shown that within 10 minutes of drinking water, the energy expenditure increases by about 30 percent! And this effect lasts for a whole hour. Another study conducted among overweight women showed that drinking just one liter of water extra per day resulted in a loss of almost 2 kilos over a period of a year. There were no other control variables here - no exercise or lifestyle changes. Just the additional drinking of one liter of water. Therefore, the results are really impressive. Also, the study revealed that just half an extra liter of water per day would cause you to burn 23 calories. This results in a massive 17,000 caloric burn over the whole year!

Natural Appetite Suppressant

We have spoken about the hunger and thirst centers located in the hypothalamus, in a different section of this book. When the stomach senses that its capacity is now full, it sends a signal to the hypothalamus, which in turn gives a feeling of "fullness" to the eater. Drinking water before meals can fool the brain into thinking that it is somewhat full, thus avoiding overeating. Because those two centers are so closely located, a person may think he or she is hungry, when thirst might be the actual issue. Drinking water also curbs unnecessary snacking between healthy meals.

Curbs Unwanted Liquid Calorie Intake

Sodas, colas, sugary drinks, fruit juices, etc. contain a large amount of sugar, which needlessly build-up problems in the body. Drinking water at regular intervals ensures that one doesn't fall prey to such liquid calories.

A Friend to Fat Burning

Water is essential to help burn fat. Without adequate water in the body, the process of metabolizing fat, called "lipolysis," cannot occur properly. The first step, called "hydrolysis," happens only in the presence of water - where the water molecules interact with triglycerides for the creation of glycerol and fatty acids. You have to drink enough water to keep this process going on smoothly and to burn fat effectively.

Workout Helper

Eating healthy and exercises are two sides of the same coin. And water helps immensely with exercise and workouts. It lubricates the joints, muscles, and tendons effectively and makes them more pliable for exercise, thus helping you on your way toward a healthy and happy body.

Nicholas Bjorn

Chapter 9 – Strength Training: A Vital Component of Your Weight Loss Journey

When you exercise and pick something you love to do, you give the best workout to your body and mind. You are also motivated further to keep eating healthy and keep moving.

Don't feel like exercising? It must be something you LOVE to do. Don't do it because your neighbor/friend/dad told you to. If you hate running or gymming or Pilates, don't do it! Pick something you love and stick to it.

Remember, you read somewhere in this book that whatever you eat is taken inside by the body for three functions: fuel, storing as fat, and rebuilding muscles, when you weight train and challenge your muscles beyond their capacity, the body's sorting behavior changes.

There's really nothing like lightweight training, so we'll leave that. A heavy workout would include a 500 lb. deadlift or 450 lb. squats. Intense bodyweight training for strength might include a handstand push up or 100 pull-ups in a minute. You get the drift.

Now when you weight train - you pick something heavy and move it against gravity for a certain number of times - your muscles break down. When you rest, eat, and sleep, they rebuild themselves in the next 48 hours. So, talking about the redirecting of calories, which happens, the body sends those calories to rebuild the broken down muscles. Also, it will direct the additional calories to burn as fuel to handle all this intense lifting activity.

So what does that mean for metabolism and weight loss? Metabolism gets a boost, and you burn calories even as you are sitting. Now, when you eat a calorie deficit and then strength train, your body gets even cleverer and stronger over time, resulting in serious weight loss without any loss in muscle mass.

Now, here's a scenario for you: You are weight training, your muscles are breaking down and need rebuilding. Because you are eating less than usual, there aren't enough calories ingested as compared to the number needed for the rebuilding process. So, what happens? Is it not worth doing all of this?

Of course not!

This is where our amazing body comes into play. Remember the "Reserve Store of Fats"? Yep. The body pulls out calories from this reserve stock and happily goes about rebuilding the muscles. You just need to keep eating enough and eat foods based on your exercise and diet goals.

Resting properly is also an important part of rebuilding muscle and keeping them strong for the next workout. This, in turn, will promote hunger at the right time, and you will eat only the right foods for your body.

Chapter 10 – Kitchen Implements and Gadgets for Healthy Cooking

Now that you are truly on your way to eating and living healthy, why not arm yourself with the right kind of tools and gadgets which will help you stick to your health plan? Here's a handy list of implements to have in your kitchen.

Steamer

Steam your vegetables for salads and veggie bowls easily.

Handheld Spiralizer

No more buying noodles and pasta from the take-out! Just use this handy spiralizer to carve your own noodles and pasta shapes at home.

Blender

A godsend for kitchens. Blend your fruit and nuts into smoothies, whip up healthy juices, and just about any dip or sauce that you like. All at the press of a button!

Nonstick Grill

This can be electric or the one you set on the stove. Grill your meats and sandwiches to perfection with the nonstick grill. Some even come with a charcoal flavor, to give you that barbeque feeling.

Rice Cooker

Another life-saving device. You can bung in your rice, measure out the water, and turn it on. By the time you're done with other activities, your rice is also done. Simply take it out and have it with whatever meats or veggies you cooked.

Nonstick Frying Pan

Takes up less oil, and you also get your meats and veggies out of it cleanly and easily.

Handheld Immersion Blender

This is different from the regular blender. With this, you plunge the blender into the foods you wish to blend. Making buttermilk, squashes, and other quick mixing drinks has never been easier!

Vegetable Peeler cum Julienne

This gadget allows you to do two things. Julienne, or cut vegetables into thin, long sticks and also peel tough veggies such as carrots and gourds.

Measuring Cups

Of course, at some point, you will want to bake and cook like a pro. These measuring cups come in very handy, having all kinds of metric conversions and quantities written clearly.

Tupperware and Prep Containers

After having worked all that hard to cook, you may have leftovers. Keep them fresh and safe inside Tupperware containers, which are microwave and dishwasher safe.

Food Processor

If you can afford this, congratulations. You've saved yourself precious hours in the kitchen. A food processor will do all these for you - chopping, dicing, slicing, shredding, mincing, pureeing, and even mixing batters and doughs! A small kitchen miracle in itself.

Nicholas Bjorn

Chapter 11 – Refrigerator Essentials for Healthy Eating

When you are surrounded by packets of chips, cans of soda, bags of pretzels, or boxes of pizza, it's really hard to even begin thinking healthily. Why not stock up your larder and refrigerator with something healthy, so that whenever you feel hungry and reach out, you will always hit something which is real food - not junk food.

Here are some foods and condiments you can keep in your fridge/pantry/freezer for continuing your healthy streak:

1. Basic Vegetables: You can store veggies like carrots, beans, celery, bell peppers, eggplant, etc. because they can stay for at least a week or so in the fridge. Just put them inside mesh bags so they can breathe properly.

2. Fruit: Apples, pears, grapes, melons, berries, citrus fruits can be stored for a good amount of time in the fridge. These make for a very healthy and tasty snack too.

3. Greens: The thing with greens is that they begin to wilt and spoil easily. So, keep your greens like kale, spinach, cilantro, and lettuce in large mesh bags or containers with drainboards underneath them. Keep them this way for a week at most.

4. Herbs: The top choices for herbs are cilantro, thyme, parsley, sage, rosemary, and dill. These can be stored fresh or in the dried form. If fresh, wrap them in dry paper and store.

5. Dried fruit: Another quick snack is dried fruit and nuts. You can store almonds, cashews, peanuts, cranberries, blueberries, dried figs, apricots, and raisins for a really long time. Use them in baking and cooking and enjoy the delicious taste. A small handful of nuts is enough to fill you up for a long time.

6. Milk: Keep a variety of milk such as almond, cashew, soy, rice, or hemp milk easily available at markets. Use them in breakfast cereal, baking, or cooking. But yes, have them sparingly.

7. Eggs: One of nature's best and cheapest nutritional hacks. When you're hungry, just boil a couple of eggs and have them with some salt and pepper. Or, scramble some eggs with butter and seasonings and have it on top of whole-wheat toast. The possibilities with eggs are limitless and equally healthy.

8. Salsa: You can either make your own salsa or buy a jar from the market. It is a delicious dip, dressing, and sauce - or simply have it with some baked sweet potato fries.

9. Mustard: Another delicious fall back option for sandwiches, stir-fries, sauces, and dressings.

10. Yeast: Store this in the active or dry form. Yeast adds a cheesy flavor to foods and is used in baking - for bread and pizza bases. Try some in your pasta and savory dishes as well.

11. Miso paste: This is a mild yet rich flavoring agent. Try it with your sauces and dips.

12. Tahini/ Nut butter: A super delicious and healthy snack would be nut butter with some crackers. Peanut and

almond butter are especially suitable for this purpose, and can also be used with sandwiches and baked stuff.

13. Soy sauce: Mostly used in Chinese cooking along with vinegar and chili sauces, you can also use soy sauce as a dressing or in salads or just one spoonful of it in a sauce - to embrace its taste and goodness.

14. Cacao powder: A fat-free and super yummy baking essential, keep some handy in your pantry or fridge to quickly whip up delicious low-calorie desserts.

For Your Freezer

1. Cooked beans: Suppose you made an extra helping of beans. Save time for the next meal by simply freezing this portion. To reuse, thaw the bag out in the fridge overnight, or run hot water over them and consume.

2. Cooked grains: Because grains take a long time to cook, it makes sense to make a larger quantity and freeze the leftovers. Storing cooked grains like rice and quinoa in the freezer will make the next meal planning a breeze.

3. Frozen vegetables: Frozen veggies such as corn, peas, carrots, cauliflower, edamame, etc. will ensure that you always have a healthy meal option to fall back on, instead of relying on take-outs.

4. Frozen fruit: Whenever there is a grocery sale, stock up on basic fruit like berries, apples, bananas, lemons, cantaloupes, grapefruit, etc. Again, a time-saving meal option.

5. Ginger and garlic: These are basic seasoning herbs and freeze very well too. Just grind together equal quantities of ginger and garlic, fry them in a little oil and when cool, put in freezer bags and freeze. Whenever you want to make a meat or veggie-based dish, just put together your frozen veggies, take the herbs from the fridge and cook them with some pre-roasted ginger and garlic and you have a meal ready in no time!

6. Corn, Rice, and Wheat Tortillas: You can quickly make wraps, tacos, and quesadillas if you have a ready store of these items in your freezer.

Chapter 12 – How to Eat Healthy Without Going Broke and Losing Your Mind

Now, eating healthy and all is great. But if you're a college student or someone who is on a tight budget or similar, it's more tempting to give in to a cheap bagel or pizza at the diner than laboriously check grocery prices and lug home bags of produce and herbs. It is even easier to just pop in a bag full of Doritos rather than get up earlier in the mornings to pack your lunch.

Yep, I hear you. But, it turns out, there are easy hacks everywhere. You can begin your healthiness quotient right now.

Love coffee and can't give it up? Cut back just one cup a day. Or bring in some homemade coffee in a flask. Another better option is to switch to green tea. Leave your tea leaves at work and bring along a hot water brewer. There is really no downside to deciding to start eating healthy. The thing is- when your body keeps getting empty calories by way of unhealthy snacks, it assumes that it will go on forever. When you suddenly start feeding it healthy stuff, it will rebel for a few days, then quickly adjust. The cravings slowly disappear, and the body starts demanding and utilizing healthy food you put into it. All this will result in a happy and sound you!

Shopping the Right Way for Health

Frequent One or Two Stores

Of course, keep an eye out on different offers, but frequent one or two places where you've been before. Check what is on sale and pick the best foods in that. Meats, veggies, fruit- doesn't matter. Pick out the best and freshest produce on display, not necessarily based on the menu you have planned for the week. Bring everything home, and THEN plan your menus. It will save you a lot of time and money.

Get Creative while Cooking

Let's say a recipe calls for green peppers, but you have yellow ones. Or it says hummus, and you forgot to buy chickpeas. There are always substitutions available. Check your pantry and fridge. Use yellow bell peppers instead of green. Or, use some miso dip instead of hummus.

Prepare Meals in Advance

It's quite easy to do this. You can chop your veggies and make batters or doughs while binge-watching your favorite shows. Even better, you can cook your chicken and veggies, portion them out and freeze them in individual serving boxes. That way, you just have to bung one in the oven before you come to work and won't have to depend on any store-bought food item for your lunch.

Buy in Bulk

Whenever possible, look out for bargains in meats and produce. Buy a whole bunch of it when on sale or discount, chop them into meal-sized portions and either freeze them immediately or cook them and then freeze.

Eat Small and Healthy Snacks

Stuff like fruit, peanut butter on crackers, carrot sticks, sprouts, popcorn, nuts are all healthy and filling snack options if you get hungry in between meals.

Eat Everything You Buy

More often than not, we go out in a rush and buy tons of food and produce and stash it all in the fridge. After about a week of hard work cooking and making meals, we fall off the wagon, and all that food keeps rotting inside the fridge. That's such a waste of money. Make it a point to stock only about a week's worth of produce and meats in your fridge and EAT ALL OF IT before you buy new food.

Learn to Cook

It doesn't necessarily have to be a Michelin rated meal. Even something as simple as scrambled eggs on toast, chicken breasts marinated and grilled, healthy low-fat sandwiches or rice wraps filled with vegetables are all great and simple starting points for meals. Pick one simple recipe and master it. Then another, and another. You can definitely learn to cook elaborate and complicated meals later on, but for now, this will do.

Nicholas Bjorn

Chapter 13 – 15 Tasty Super Food Smoothies Recipes

The following recipes all contain superfoods and are another alternative as a way of making sure that you get all you need in your diet. With the smoothies, simply add all the ingredients to your blender, whiz them up and enjoy!

Peanut Butter Power Shake

- 1 scoop of whey protein powder, chocolate flavored
- 1 tbsp. organic or natural peanut butter
- ½ banana
- 1 cup of almond milk
- Ice cubes

Dark Chocolate Shake

- 1 scoop whey protein , chocolate flavored
- 1 cup almond milk
- 2 ½ tbsp. cacao powder
- 2 ice cubes

CHIA Green Smoothie

- 1 scoop whey protein vanilla
- 1 tbsp. chia seeds
- 1 cup spinach
- 1 cup almond milk
- 1 banana
- water/ice

The Winter Mint Chocolate Shake

- 1 scoop whey protein , chocolate or chocolate mint
- 1 cup almond milk
- 1/2 cup arctic zero mint chocolate
- 1 drop peppermint extract
- 2 ice cubes

Green Spinach-Apple-Mango Yogurt Smoothie

- 3/4 cup plain 0% Greek yogurt
- 1/2 bunch spinach
- 1 apple
- 1/2 cup mango chunks
- 1 cup ice/water

Anti-Aging Kiwi-Blueberry Smoothie

- 1/2 scoop whey protein, vanilla
- 1/2 cup 0% plain Greek yogurt
- 1 cup flax milk
- 2 kiwi
- 1/2 cup blueberries
- 2 ice cubes

Berry Banana Smoothie

- 1 scoop whey protein, vanilla
- 1 cup flax milk
- 1/2 cup blackberries
- 1/2 banana
- 1/2 cup raspberries
- 1/2 cup strawberries
- 2 ice cubes

Peach-Mango Yogurt Smoothie

- 1 Cup plain 0% Greek yogurt
- 1 peach
- 1 cup mango chunks
- 1/4 tsp. cinnamon
- 1 cup ice

The Lean Muscle Mochaccino

- 1 scoop whey protein, mocha cappuccino
- 1.5 cups flax milk
- 2.5 tbsp. cacao powder
- 2 ice cubes

Orange Creamsicle Smoothie

- 1 scoop whey protein, orange creamsicle
- 1 medium orange
- 1 cup almond milk
- 1/2 cup orange juice
- 1 cup water/ice

Liquid Breakfast Smoothie

- 3/4 cup plain 0% Greek yogurt
- 1/2 banana
- 1/4 cup rolled oats
- 1 cup strawberries
- 1 cup water/Ice

Banana Nut Shake

- 1 scoop vanilla whey protein
- 1 cup almond milk
- 1 large banana
- 3 tbsp. organic peanut butter
- water/ice

Strawberry Shortcake Smoothie

- 3/4 cup plain 0% Greek yogurt
- 1 cup strawberries
- 1/2 cup rolled oats
- 1 tsp vanilla extract
- water/ice

Mango Pineapple Shake

- 1 scoop vanilla whey protein
- 1/2 cup mango chunks
- 1/2 cup pineapple chunks
- 1 cup almond Milk

Creamy Chocolate Avocado Smoothie

- 1 scoop chocolate whey protein
- 1/2 small avocado
- 3/4 banana
- 1 1/2 cup ice/Water

Chapter 14 – 5 Tasty Super Food Soup Recipes

Green Superfood Soup

Ingredients:

- 185 g broccoli
- 2 leeks sliced
- 1 onion roughly diced
- ½ teaspoon garlic oil or minced garlic
- 1 cup green split peas – soaked for 1 hour, rinsed
- 310 g medium cauliflower
- 9-10 g dry wakame seaweed – soaked for 10 min, roughly chopped
- 80 g kale – roughly chopped
- ½ cup stock
- pinch sea salt
- pepper
- ¼ tsp thyme
- enough water to cover
- Oil for cooking

- Coconut cream

Instructions:

1. Heat up the oil in a large pan
2. Cook the onions and leeks until they are brown
3. Add all other ingredients, add the stock and enough water to cover the vegetables
4. Simmer for about 1 hour over a low heat, or until the split peas are soft
5. Blend in the blender to make a thick soup
6. Add in some coconut cream and water to bring it to the consistency you like
7. Season with salt and pepper

Carrot and Turmeric Soup

Ingredients:

- 500 g carrots
- 2 garlic cloves
- 1 onion, white
- 1 tbsp. coconut oil
- 2 tsp turmeric
- 1 tbsp. fresh ginger
- 400 ml stock
- 150 ml water
- Salt and pepper
- 1 lime

Instructions:

1. Chop the carrots into pieces about an inch in size and peel the garlic; set aside
2. Cut the onion into small bits and fry over a medium heat with a pinch of salt and 1 tbsp. oil
3. Add the ginger and turmeric and cook for 30 seconds, stirring
4. Crush the garlic and add it in, stir and add the carrots

5. Roast for a few minutes before adding the stock

6. Use a blender to blend the soup until smooth – add more water if needed

7. Add another inch of salt, pepper and squeeze the juice in from the lime

Dairy-Free Creamy Avocado Soup

Ingredients:

- 3 ripe avocado, peeled, pitted and chopped
- 2 cups plain dairy-free yogurt
- ⅓ cup cashews
- ⅓ cup finely chopped fresh cilantro
- ⅓ cup Vidalia onion, chopped
- 1 Tbsp. white balsamic vinegar
- 1 cup green tea, brewed and chilled
- 1 tsp. sea salt
- ¼ tsp. freshly ground white pepper
- 2 chives, finely chopped

Instructions:

1. Blend the avocado, yoghurt, cilantro, almonds, onion, vinegar, green tea, pepper and sea salt until smooth
2. Transfer into a bowl and cover; refrigerate for 2 hours
3. Serve chilled and garnished with chopped chives

Spicy Chicken and Quinoa Soup

Ingredients:

- 2 tbsp. extra virgin olive oil
- 1 cup diced onion
- 2 garlic cloves, chopped
- 2 tomatoes, peeled and diced
- 2 carrots, peeled and chopped
- 1 tsp of paprika
- 2 tsp of cumin
- 2 cups of white meat from 2 baked skinless and shredded organic chicken breasts
- 2 cups of filtered water
- 4 cups low sodium organic chicken broth
- 2 cups of fresh or frozen peas
- 2 cups cooked quinoa
- 4 tbsp. finely chopped parsley
- 3 tbsp. finely chopped cilantro
- 1 tsp kosher salt
- Freshly ground black pepper

Instructions:

1. Heat up the olive oil in a large soup pot
2. Add the onions, garlic and sauté until translucent, about 5 minutes
3. Add the tomato, carrots, cumin and pepper, cook for a father 5 minutes, stirring
4. Add the water and broth, turn the heat up to high and bring to a boil
5. Add the peas, quinoa, herbs and chicken, season with salt and peeper
6. Reduce heat and simmer for 25 minutes
7. Serve hot with a diced avocado

To Bake Chicken Breasts

1. Preheat the oven to 350° F
2. Rub olive oil over the chicken and season with salt and pepper
3. Place in a foil lined baking sheet, skin side up and bake for 40 to 45 minutes
4. Remove and allow it to cool off before taking the skin off and shredding it

Slow Cooker Superfood Soup

Ingredients:

- 2 cups sliced carrots
- 1 large sweet potato, cut into 1/2" cubes
- 1 cup fresh or frozen green beans
- 1/2 cup fresh cilantro, chopped
- 1 small onion, diced
- 1 clove garlic, minced
- 2 (15 ounce) cans black beans, drained and rinsed
- 1/2 teaspoon crushed red pepper flakes
- 1/2 teaspoon black pepper
- 1 teaspoon chili powder
- 1 teaspoon cumin
- Kosher or sea salt to taste
- 2 cups vegetable juice (I used R.W. Knudsen, Organic Very Veggie Juice, no sugar added)
- 2 cups vegetable broth, low-sodium

Instructions:

1. Mix all the ingredients together in your slow cooker, cover and cook it for about 6-8 hours on low, or until the

vegetables have gone tender. If you want, you can add in a tbsp. of low fat cheddar cheese

You can sauté onion in 1 tbsp. olive oil for 5 minutes and then add the garlic and sauté for a further 1 minute before adding them to the slow cooker. You can also add in 2 cups of coarsely chopped kale about 5 minutes before the end of cooking

Chapter 15 – 6 Yummy and Healthy One-Bowl Meals

Quinoa and Chicken Burrito Bowl with Green Sauce

Ingredients:

For the quinoa:

- 1.5 cups pre washed quinoa
- ¾ tsp salt

For the chicken:

- 2 pounds chicken tenderloin or boneless chicken pounded to ½ inch thickness
- 5 tbsp. extra virgin olive oil
- 2 tsp honey
- 4 garlic cloves, minced
- ½ tsp ground black pepper
- 1 tbsp. lime zest (from two limes)
- 1-1/4 tsp chili powder

- ½ tsp coriander (fresh or dry)
- ¼ tsp dried oregano
- Salt: As per taste

For the green sauce:

- 1 jalapeno chili pepper, seeded and chopped
- 1 cup cilantro leaves
- 2 garlic cloves, chopped
- ¼ cup sour cream
- ½ cup mayonnaise
- 1 tbsp. fresh lime juice
- 2 tbsp. extra virgin olive oil
- Salt and pepper - As per taste

Instructions:

The Chicken

1. Mix all the ingredients except the chicken breasts in a large freezer bag. Close it and thoroughly mix all the ingredients together.

2. Add the chicken breasts into the marinade and mix until every piece is evenly coated with it. Seal the bag and put it inside the fridge (preferably in a bowl) and let it marinate for at least 6 hours or overnight.

3. When it is fully marinated, take the bag out of the fridge.

4. Clean your grill and put it onto preheat. Spray it with a nonstick cooking spray or lightly coat the grill with oil until it is well oiled.

5. Take the chicken pieces out and lay them on the grill. Slowly grill them for two or three minutes on each side and transfer to a plate. Cut them into bite-sized pieces.

The Quinoa

1. Mix the quinoa, salt, and around two and a half cups of water in a saucepan.

2. Let it come to a boil, then reduce the flame and cover.

3. Cook for ten to fifteen minutes until the quinoa absorbs water and gets cooked. When done, take it out in a bowl and keep aside.

The Sauce

1. Mix all the sauce ingredients in a blender and combine to make a smooth puree. Taste and check for seasonings. If you wish to make it in advance, you can put this sauce into a bowl and refrigerate it until you want to eat.

How to Assemble

Get your quinoa bowl in front of you. Put the grilled chicken on top, and pour the sauce over it. If you wish, you can add additional toppings like tomatoes, diced pumpkin, carrots, or celery.

French Lentil Salad with Goat Cheese

Ingredients:

- 1 cup French lentils (or any other lentils)
- 3 ounces goat cheese
- 3 cups chicken broth
- 1 large carrot, finely chopped
- 2 celery stalks, finely chopped
- 1 small bay leaf
- 1 tsp fresh thyme
- 3 tbsp. parsley, chopped
- 2 garlic cloves, chopped
- 1 tsp mustard
- 1 tsp honey
- Salt: As per taste

Instructions:

1. Wash and rinse the lentils well.

2. Mix lentils, chicken broth, and bay leaf in a saucepan. Let it boil for a few minutes, then simmer them over low heat until the lentils are soft and tender. This may take about 20 to 25 minutes.

3. After this, remove the bay leaf and drain the water from the lentils.

4. In a bowl, mix together all ingredients except the goat cheese.

5. When the lentils are cool, add them to the bowl, adjust seasonings and toss to combine well.

6. Just before eating, crumble the goat cheese over the salad and serve. You may wish to serve the salad with fresh iceberg lettuce leaves.

Thai Chicken Soup with Rice Noodles

Ingredients:

- 4 cups chicken broth
- ½ cup shallots, thinly sliced
- 2 tbsp. Thai green curry paste
- 1 tbsp. vegetable oil
- 1 tbsp. fresh ginger, minced
- 2 tbsp. fish sauce
- 1 can coconut milk
- 4 heaped tsp brown sugar
- 2 tbsp. fresh lime juice
- ½ tsp turmeric
- 1 pack rice noodles

Instructions:

1. Heat the oil in a medium-sized saucepan or soup pot.
2. Add the ginger and shallots and cook for a few minutes, stirring constantly. Don't let the ginger burn.
3. Mix in the curry paste and cook for a minute.

4. Add the chicken broth, coconut milk, brown sugar, fish sauce, turmeric, and lime juice. Add salt if you wish to.

5. Bring to a simmer and gently cook for about five to six minutes.

6. While this is happening, make the rice noodles according to the instructions on the package.

How to Assemble

Adjust seasonings in the soup. Pour the soup over the rice noodles and gently give it a mix. You can serve this with cilantro or celery, and chopped scallions. You may also drizzle some Sriracha sauce over it.

Cauliflower Fried Rice

Ingredients:

- 2 lb. cauliflower
- 4 to 5 tbsp. vegetable oil
- 2 large eggs, beaten
- 2 scallions, chopped finely
- 3 garlic cloves, chopped
- 1 tbsp. freshly chopped ginger
- 4 tbsp. soy sauce
- 1 cup peas and carrots (frozen peas and carrots also work)
- ¼ tsp red pepper flakes
- 1 tsp honey
- 1 tsp rice vinegar
- 1 tsp sesame oil
- ¼ cup chopped cashews/ almonds/ peanuts
- Salt: As per taste

Instructions:

1. Grate the cauliflower, either by hand or in a food processor.

2. Heat the vegetable oil in a large skillet or cast iron pan.

3. Add the eggs and salt and keep cooking until the eggs are scrambled and cooked. Keep aside on a small plate. Carefully wipe the pan.

4. Again, add about 3 tbsp. of vegetable oil to the pan and keep it at medium heat. Add in the scallions, garlic, and ginger and cook gently.

5. Mix in the grated cauliflower, red pepper, soy sauce, honey, and salt. Keep stirring.

6. Then add the peas and carrots and keep cooking until the cauliflower is soft and the vegetables are tender.

7. After five minutes, add the rice vinegar, sesame oil, and nuts.

8. After about two minutes, add the eggs. Keep tasting and adjusting the seasoning.

9. Take off the fire and serve right away with a dash of soy sauce on top.

Thai Shrimp and Quinoa

Ingredients:

- 1 pound raw jumbo shrimp (cleaned, deveined and tail off)
- 2 cups chicken stock
- 1 and a 1/2 cups quinoa, uncooked
- 1 cup coconut milk
- 1 tbsp. coconut or any other oil
- 1 tbsp. fish sauce
- ½ cup small onion, chopped
- ½ tsp sesame oil
- 1 each, red and yellow bell peppers, chopped
- 2 medium carrots, julienned
- ½ tsp ground ginger
- Salt: As per taste
- 3 cloves minced garlic
- ¼ tsp red pepper flakes
- ½ a lime, chopped

Instructions:

1. Take a large cast-iron pan or skillet and heat the oil for a couple of minutes.

2. Add the fish sauce and sesame oil and stir.

3. After a couple of minutes, add the bell pepper, carrots, and onion and ginger. Add some salt at this stage.

4. Cook for four or five minutes until the vegetables become tender.

5. Now add the garlic and cook for another minute.

6. Add the coconut milk, quinoa, and chicken stock. Mix well, cover, and cook for almost 15 minutes until the quinoa is fully cooked.

7. Once done, remove the lid and add the shrimp to the mixture.

8. Adjust seasoning and add pepper flakes to it. Cover and cook for five to six minutes until the shrimp is translucent and cooked.

9. Serve hot with wedges of lime and a dash of cilantro on top.

Ratatouille Rice

Ingredients:

- 1 tbsp. olive oil
- 1 medium onion, diced
- 3 cloves minced garlic
- 1 medium zucchini, diced
- ½ eggplant, diced
- 1/8 tsp ground black pepper
- ½ tsp dried oregano
- ¼ tsp red pepper flakes
- 1 red bell pepper, diced
- 2 small tomatoes, diced
- 1 cup white rice
- 1 cup vegetable broth

Instructions:

1. Take a skillet and warm the olive oil for a minute.

2. Add in the onion with a bit of salt, and cook until it becomes translucent and tender.

3. Add the garlic and cook until it gives off a nice aroma.

4. Now add the eggplant, zucchini, black pepper, oregano, pepper flakes, some salt, and stir. Cook this for about a minute or so.

5. Then mix in the tomatoes and bell pepper and cook until the tomato starts releasing oil and liquid around it.

6. Lastly, add the white rice and vegetable broth. Stir until combined and bring to a boil.

7. After a couple of minutes, simmer the mixture and cover and cook for about 18 minutes, until the rice is completely cooked. If you feel the rice is sticking to the bottom, add some more broth.

8. Check seasonings and add pepper, salt, herbs as desired. Serve this healthy dish hot from the stove, garnished with cilantro and basil.

Chapter 16 – Sweet Endings: Lip Smacking Healthy Desserts

So you thought desserts are the work of the Devil, full of rich and sinful things that you eat just once and repent at leisure? Do not fret. Here are some absolutely delicious desserts for you to indulge in, without going off the health wagon.

Avocado Chocolate Mousse with Summer Fruit

Ingredients:

- 4 ripe avocado
- ¼ cup coconut milk
- 4 tbsp. dark cocoa powder
- 3 tbsp. honey
- 2 ounces dark chocolate, melted (70 percent or more cocoa)
- 2 tsp vanilla extract
- 1/8 tsp salt
- Coconut whipped cream, strawberries, blueberries, and other summer fruit, chopped

Instructions:

1. Peel and pit the avocado and put them inside a food processor.

2. Blend until well combined and creamy.

3. Mix in the cocoa, honey, milk, vanilla, chocolate, and salt. Keep blending until they mix properly. Taste at this point and add more honey if desired. The mixture should be completely creamy at the end of this.

4. Serving: Take out into pretty bowls and top with coconut cream or layer it with summer fruit such as berries, mangoes, even nuts and add a few nuts for extra crunch.

Raspberry Vegan Cheesecake

Ingredients:

For walnut crust

- 1 cup walnuts
- 3 dates (Mejdool or similar), pitted
- ½ tbsp. coconut oil
- ¼ tsp sea salt

For the raspberry layer

- 12 ounces frozen raspberries
- ½ tsp fresh lemon juice
- 2 tbsp. maple syrup
- 2 tbsp. chia seeds

Instructions:

1. Blend together the walnuts, salt, dates, and coconut oil in a food processor until the mixture turns crumbly.
2. Line an 8" by 4" loaf pan with parchment paper. You can also butter it beforehand. Press the crust onto the bottom and freeze until the next layer is ready.

3. Blend together the thawed raspberries, maple syrup, lemon juice, and chia seeds. The mixture should be smooth; no bits should be visible. Pour this mixture over the frozen walnut crust and smooth it out. Freeze this for at least four hours.

4. When you are ready to serve this dessert, take the cake out of the freezer and let it thaw for about twenty minutes.

5. Lift it out carefully from the pan. Slice into as many slices as you would like. Garnish with a sprig of mint for extra flavor.

Cinnamon Baked Pears

Ingredients:

- 2 pears, washed, cored and cut in half
- 1 tsp cinnamon
- 1 tsp maple syrup
- Pumpkin spice granola and coconut cream for toppings

Instructions:

1. Before doing anything, preheat the oven to 350 degrees.
2. Take a baking sheet and place the pears on it. It should stand straight on the paper. Or you may cut into any shape you desire or even bite-sized pieces.
3. Sprinkle it evenly with the maple syrup and cinnamon. Bake this for about 25 minutes.
4. Cool them and top with either the granola or any other nuts or berries and enjoy.

Healthy Peanut Butter Fudge

Ingredients:

- 2 cups finely shredded coconut
- 1 cup creamy peanut butter
- ½ cup coconut oil
- 4 tbsp maple syrup
- 1 pinch sea salt
- 1 tsp vanilla extract
- Toppings: peanuts, coconut flakes, nuts, etc.

Instructions:

1. First, line a 9" by 5" loaf tin with parchment paper.
2. Add the desiccated coconut to a food processor and blend on high speed until the mixture becomes creamy. Scrape down the sides and keep aside.
3. Add the peanut butter and coconut oil and blend one again at high speed.
4. Once done, mix in the maple syrup one tablespoon at a time. Check for sweetness and add until the desired level is reached. Don't add too much because then the coconut mixture with seize and you won't be able to work with it.

5. Add sea salt and vanilla extract and mix well.

6. Transfer this to the loaf pan or tin and spread it evenly all over. At this point, you can also add some crunch on top by putting nuts or flakes.

7. Now freeze this until it becomes firm. Take a knife and run it through hot water and cut the mixture into even squares. This will give you about twenty squares.

8. Serve immediately and enjoy it. You can also store these in the freezer for up to a month.

No-Bake Brownie Energy Bites

Ingredients:

- ½ cup each walnuts and almonds
- 1 cup dates, chopped
- 1/3 cup plus 2 tbsp. unsweetened cocoa powder
- ½ cup shredded coconut flakes

Instructions:

1. Grind together the walnuts and almonds in a food processor. The mixture should form a dough.
2. Mix in the dates, coconut, cocoa, and a pinch of salt and incorporate it well into the dough.
3. Now, lightly grease your palms with coconut oil or use saran wrap to make balls out of the dough.
4. Roll these into the remaining coconut flakes or use corn flakes or almonds to coat the balls. Put them inside the fridge for a little while. Take them out and serve.

Apple Crumble

Ingredients:

- 5 apples, Granny Smith or similar
- ½ cup low-fat butter
- 3 and a half tbsp. flour
- ½ cup honey or maple syrup
- 1 lime
- 1 small stick cinnamon
- 1 tbsp. sugar
- Coconut cream: Optional

Instructions:

1. Preheat the oven to 180 degrees Celsius.
2. For the topping, take the butter in a plate and sift flour over it.
3. Add the honey. Mix these by hand until you get a crumbly mixture.
4. Peel the apples and cut them in half or bite-sized pieces. Place these in an ovenproof bowl.

5. Squeeze the lime over them and shake so that it is distributed equally, and the apples are not discolored. Sprinkle the one tablespoon sugar over them. Put in the stick of cinnamon over this.

6. When ready to go inside the oven, sprinkle the topping you just made over the apples. Bake for about 40 minutes, till the apple crumble turns golden brown.

7. Serve either hot or cold with coconut cream.

Yogurt Cocktail

Ingredients:

- 1 and a half cups yogurt or curd
- ½ cup plums
- 4 medium strawberries
- ¼ cup pineapple
- 4 tbsp. honey
- ½ tsp vanilla extract
- ½ cup non-dairy cream or coconut cream
- A few cornflakes- different flavorings

Instructions:

1. Chop the fruit into bite-sized pieces and put the mix in a big microwaveable bowl. Add some honey and microwave them on high for a minute.

2. Combine the yogurt, remaining honey, and vanilla in a bowl.

3. Add the coconut cream and mix well. Either put it in the fridge or strain through a muslin cloth to get rid of excess water and then put it in the fridge, depending on how you like the consistency.

4. Take the fruit bowl out of the microwave.

5. Layer the fruit one by one alternating with the yogurt mixture in a large glass bowl. For garnishing, use cornflakes or coconut flakes or any nuts of your choice.

Quick Coffee Dessert

Ingredients:

- 2 eggs
- ½ cup ground sugar or maple syrup
- A pinch of salt
- 1 tbsp. instant coffee
- 1 cup whipping cream or nondairy cream
- 2 tbsp. castor sugar
- 1 tsp vanilla extract
- ¼ tsp almond essence

Instructions:

1. Put the eggs, salt, and sugar in a bowl and beat with a hand mixer at high speed. The mixture will become lemony and fluffy.

2. Add the coffee and beat for a few more minutes. Keep this aside.

3. In another bowl, take the cream and sugar and whip until soft peaks form. It shouldn't be too runny or too stiff. Gently stir in the essences.

4. Fold the egg mixture into the cream and combine gently, making sure you don't lose the aeration.

5. Pour into individual glasses and freeze until you are ready to eat.

6. When serving, take the glasses out and let them sit for about ten minutes or so before digging in. If you wish, garnish with mint leaves.

Simple Rice Pudding

Ingredients:

- ½ cup rice washed and soaked in ½ cup low-fat milk
- 5 and a half cups low fat milk
- ½ cup sugar or honey
- Almonds: Blanched and slivered, a few
- Rosewater: A few drops
- Pistachios: A few

Instructions:

1. Blend the rice and milk, such that it becomes an absolutely smooth paste.
2. Take the other milk in a vessel and boil it. Pour the rice-milk paste and sugar or honey into it and continuously stir it on a low flame until the mixture thickens. Simmer for a while.
3. Take it off the fire.
4. Add the almonds and pistachios, along with the rose water and mix well. Pour into glasses or bowls and chill well. Serve with a glass of cold milk, if so desired.

Rich Chocolate Slices

Ingredients:

- ½ cup butter or low-fat margarine
- 2 tbsp. honey
- 4 and a half tbsp. cocoa
- 225 grams semi-sweet biscuits
- 2 tbsp. raisins
- 2 tbsp. chopped mixed nuts

Instructions:

1. Mix the honey, cocoa, and butter in a pan and put it on a gentle heat. You will need to keep a watch over it and remove it as soon as the butter melts.//
2. Mix the ingredients of the pan well and keep aside.
3. Meanwhile, crush the biscuits in a clean bag with a rolling pin or blend in a processor. You can do the same with the nuts. Keep aside.
4. When the butter mixture cools down, add the biscuit and nut mixture to it. Mix well. The final consistency should be crumbly, yet it should hold well when you compress it.

5. Grease a small cake tin with oil or butter and pour this mixture into it. Leave it inside the fridge to set.

6. For serving, let it rest on the countertop or dip the tin into hot water for a few seconds and invert it over a plate. Cut into slices and serve with fresh fruit on the side.

Nicholas Bjorn

Conclusion

If it wasn't clear from the beginning, stop chasing the latest diet trend and focus on the healthy weight loss and super foods in this book. Know that you can eat normally and still lose weight.

Your next step is to follow the strategies and recipes listed in this book. Apply what you have just learned. Take action and be consistent! The best thing you can do to lose weight and be healthier is to eat right.

Now, I would love to hear what you think! Please let me know if you enjoyed this book or what I could improve on. You can do that by leaving a review on Amazon. I'll be looking for your reviews when I come back to add more content my book. Thank you in advance!

Thank you, and good luck!

Nicholas Bjorn

Nicholas Bjorn

FREE E-BOOKS SENT WEEKLY

Join North Star Readers Book Club
And Get Exclusive Access To The Latest Kindle Books in
Health, Fitness, Weight Loss and Much More...

TO GET YOU STARTED HERE IS YOUR FREE E-BOOK:

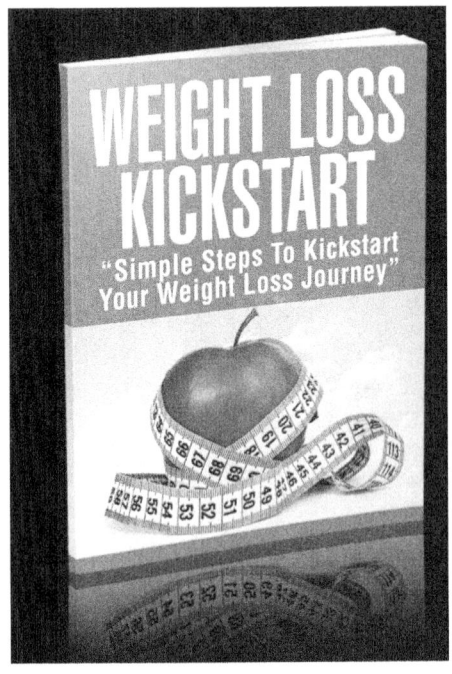

Visit to Sign Up Today!
www.northstarreaders.com/weight-loss-kick-start

References

https://www.healthline.com/nutrition/top-10-evidence-based-health-benefits-of-coconut-oil#section10

https://www.ausnaturalcare.com.au/health/lifestyle/lifestyle/food/goji-berries-real-superfood

https://www.healthline.com/nutrition/11-proven-health-benefits-of-garlic

www.webmd.com

www.self.com

www.mayoclinic.com

www.nerdfitness.com

www.buzzfeed.com

www.tasty.co

www.healthline.com

www.jamieoliver.com

GOOD NUTRITION IS IMPORTANT – THIS IS A FACT.

BUT HOW DO YOU REALLY GET STARTED TO ACHIEVING IT? PEOPLE SAY IT BEGINS WITH A BALANCED DIET, BUT HOW EXACTLY DO YOU ACHIEVE THAT BALANCE?

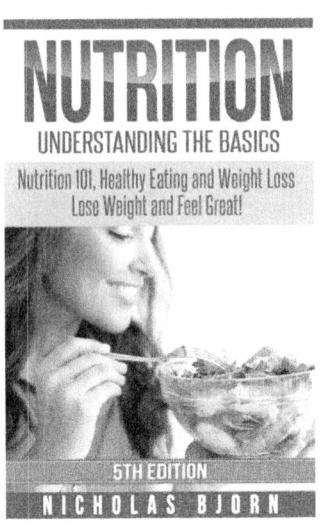

If you are lost in the world of calories and kilojoules, this book is the perfect reference to help you! The contents of this book will help you focus on what's important while getting rid of all the unnecessary fluff about dieting and healthy living that are just bound to confuse you.

Here is what this book has in store for you:
- Nutrition defined and simplified
- Dietary guidelines made easy to follow
- Nutrition labels made understandable
- Vitamins and minerals explained
- Fat-burning foods enumerated
- Meal planning and recipes made doable

Start reaping the benefits of eating healthy and living healthy! You can get started today.

Visit to Order Your Copy Today!
https://www.amazon.com/dp/1519485492

DO YOU WANT TO KNOW HOW YOU CAN LOSE WEIGHT AND BUILD MUSCLE FAST, STARTING RIGHT NOW? THIS BOOK WILL LET YOU IN ON THE SECRET!

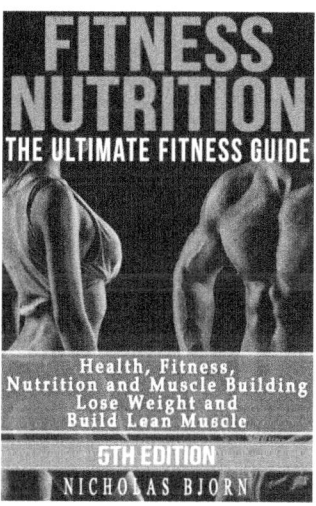

Everyone knows how important it is to maintain a healthy physique. Often, achieving the ideal body requires you to lose weight and build lean muscle. But how do you do that? To become physically fit, you need to have the knowledge necessary to get you on your way and the motivation required to keep you going.

Here's what this book has in store for you:
- Learn how your body uses calories and what role carbohydrates play in your weight
- Discover which foods contain good fats and lean protein that could benefit your body
- Determine what your meal frequency and caloric intake should be
- Know which exercises you should do to get that toned and sculpted look

With the knowledge you will gain from this book, you will be on your way to getting the amazing body that you want!

Visit to Order Your Copy Today!
https://www.amazon.com/dp/1514832968

Printed in Great Britain
by Amazon